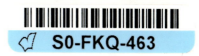

World Food Supply

This is a volume in the Arno Press collection

World Food Supply

Advisory Editor
D. Gale Johnson

Editorial Board
Charles M. Hardin
Kenneth H. Parsons

See last pages of this volume for a complete list of titles.

Efficient Use of Food Resources in the United States

RAYMOND P. CHRISTENSEN

ARNO PRESS

A New York Times Company

New York — 1976

Editorial Supervision: MARIE STARECK

———◆———

Reprint Edition 1976 by Arno Press Inc.

Reprinted from a copy in
  The University of Illinois Library

WORLD FOOD SUPPLY
ISBN for complete set: 0-405-07766-1
See last pages of this volume for titles.

Manufactured in the United States of America

———◆———

Library of Congress Cataloging in Publication Data

Christensen, Raymond Peter, 1914-
    Efficient use of food resources in the United States.

    (World food supply)
    Reprint of the 1948 ed. published by the U. S. Govt.
Print. Off., Washington, which was issued as Technical
bulletin no. 963 of the U. S. Dept. of Agriculture.
    Bibliography: p.
    1. Food supply--United States. 2. Food consump-
tion--United States. 3. Diet--United States. I. Ti-
tle. II. Series. III. Series: United States. Dept.
of Agriculture. Technical bulletin ; no. 963.
HD9005.6.C48   338.1'9'73   75-26300
ISBN 0-405-07772-6

TECHNICAL BULLETIN No. 963   October, 1948

Efficient Use of Food Resources
in the United States

By
RAYMOND P. CHRISTENSEN
Agricultural Economist
Bureau of Agricultural Economics

UNITED STATES DEPARTMENT OF AGRICULTURE, WASHINGTON, D. C.

Technical Bulletin No. 963 • *October 1948*

UNITED STATES
DEPARTMENT OF AGRICULTURE
WASHINGTON, D. C.

Efficient Use of Food Resources in the United States [1]

By RAYMOND P. CHRISTENSEN

Agricultural Economist, Bureau of Agricultural Economics [2]

CONTENTS

THE LONG-TERM FOOD PROBLEM

Food production and consumption in the United States reached record levels during the war years. The level of food production averaged one-third higher in 1942–45 than in 1935–39 and was still higher in 1946 and 1947. The expansion during the war was as great as that which took place during the 30 years from 1909 to 1939 and more than twice as great as the expansion during the First World War, or during the interwar period.

Productive capacity of agriculture was increased gradually during the interwar years by improvements in farm technology which made

[1] Received for publication April 13, 1948. The work represented by this publication was supported in part by Bankhead-Jones special research funds.

[2] The assistance provided by the comments and suggestions of Ronald L. Mighell of the Bureau of Agricultural Economics and Esther F. Phipard of the Bureau of Human Nutrition and Home Economics is gratefully acknowledged. This study is a revision and expansion of the earlier report by Raymond P. Christensen, Using Resources to Meet Food Needs, Bur. Agr. Econ., 71 pp. 1943. (Processed.)

1

possible higher rates of output per farm worker and per acre of land But this increased capacity did not bring the increased production that it might, because of unfavorable weather in some years and the failure of the demand for farm products to increase, particularly after 1929.   Not until the wartime demands for food made the newly developed methods of production highly profitable were they utilized fully to expand production.   Even then, expansion was limited by wartime scarcities of labor, machinery, and other materials.   But the removal of these limitations and the inevitable additional advances in farm technology will make possible further increases in food production.

The total volume of food consumption in the United States increased gradually, at about the same rate as total population, from 1909 to 1939, but it has increased more rapidly during the last few years.

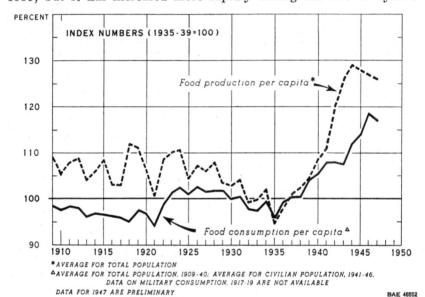

FIGURE 1.—Food production and food consumption per capita in the United States, 1909–47.

Even so, this increase has not been so rapid as the increase in production.   Per capita consumption of food products averaged 10 percent higher in the 1942–45 war years and 18 percent higher in 1946 than it did in 1935–39.   However, food production per capita averaged 27 percent higher during the last 5 years than it did immediately before the war (fig. 1).

Increased consumption, civilian and military, caused by population growth and higher per capita rates of consumption, absorbed about half of the expansion in food production between 1935–39 and 1942–45 and nearly three-fourths of the expansion between the prewar period and 1946.   The remainder went into increased exports, including lend-lease and military shipments for foreign feeding.   Imports of food products have remained relatively stable for the last several years, but exports during the last 5 years were about four times as great as immediately before the war (fig. 2).   Exports of food products were 2.8 percent and imports 6.8 percent of total food production in the United States in 1935–39; but since 1941, exports have exceeded imports.

A relatively high level of food consumption, as compared with that of prewar years, will be necessary to make full use of agricultural production capacity in the period ahead. For example, if per capita food production continues at the same rate as in recent years and if foreign trade returns to prewar levels, enough food would be available for per capita consumption to average 27 percent higher in the years ahead than it did in 1935–39. Exports of food products may remain high for the next several years. But if they decline to prewar levels by 1955 and if production equals the recent wartime vol-

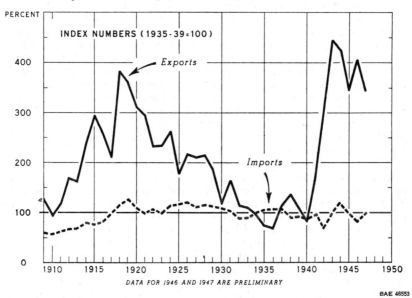

FIGURE 2.—Physical volume of exports and imports of food products, United States, 1909–47.

ume, enough food would be available for per capita consumption of the expected population to average 15 percent higher than it did immediately before the war.

Total demand for food products has been large enough in recent years to provide market outlets at relatively high prices for all that could be produced. This general situation can be expected to continue if domestic demand remains high. A reduction in foreign demand to prewar levels of course would mean some reduction in total demand for food products. For example, the per capita supply of food available for domestic consumption would have been about 6 percent higher in 1946 if foreign trade had averaged the same as before the war. If employment and incomes remain at high levels, however, this food supply probably could be marketed at prices not much lower than those in 1946. But adjustments in the production and consumption, particularly for some products, would be necessary if the most efficient use of resources in supplying consumer demand is to be made. These adjustments can be ascertained at least approximately by comparing recent production with national requirements for food products with a high level of per capita consumption, as in 1946 or 1947.

On the other hand, a return of demand conditions similar to those that prevailed just before the war, which would accompany a general decline in employment and incomes, would mean that a per capita food supply at recent levels could not be sold except at prices much lower than those of recent years. Surplus production would result, in the sense that the total food supply could not be marketed at prices profitable to all producers. Physical needs and wants for food would not be reduced significantly, however, and it still would be desirable from a national standpoint to utilize resources available for food production to satisfy needs and wants as fully as possible (26).[3]

Considerable attention has been given to methods of expanding food consumption in a period when demand is not great enough to provide market outlets at profitable prices for all the available food. They usually include the objective of improving diets that are inadequate from a nutritional standpoint. Of course, better nutrition is a desirable national objective regardless of general economic conditions, but diets usually are most inadequate when incomes and purchasing power decline. It also is obvious that measures put into effect to expand food consumption and provide better diets should result in greater satisfaction of food preferences and tastes, so far as possible with the available food-production capacity.

What adjustments in production and consumption of food products would be necessary in the period ahead to provide better diets and at the same time satisfy tastes and preferences as fully as possible? This is the central question under study here. The analytical procedure followed may be described briefly as follows:

1. Estimates are made of the increases in national consumption of food nutrients (calories, protein, minerals, and vitamins) that would be necessary if all diets that are below a specified level of adequacy were raised to such a level. Consumption of food products could be changed in many ways to supply these additional nutrients.

2. Changes in food production in the past are examined next, to decide how supplies of food products and nutrients can be increased in the future.

3. The relative efficiencies of food products as sources of food nutrients are examined in detail to find how the total supplies of nutrients from the resources available for use in food production can be increased by shifting resources to produce more of the products that provide larger outputs of nutrients per unit of resources. These data provide a basis for deciding how the nutritional requirements of a population can be met even if it is not possible to increase the supply of resources available for food production.

4. Possible changes in the total volume of food production in the future are then considered, to indicate what rates of per capita consumption may be possible. Information about food preferences is examined to decide what changes in consumption could be made to supply needs for additional nutrients in the kinds of products that would satisfy preferences most fully. Methods of achieving these consumption changes are considered briefly.

---

[3] Italic numbers in parentheses refer to Literature Cited, p. 67.

5. Finally, the adjustments in national production of food products that would be necessary to supply better diets made up of the kinds of food that people prefer are indicated by comparing present production with national requirements if such consumption changes are to be made.

The adjustments in production and consumption of food products that are described in this study relate mainly to the years beyond the foreign recovery period when per capita supplies of food may average much larger than they have in the past. But information is also presented to show how resources can be used most effectively in periods of food shortages or greatly increased food needs. For example, the data showing the outputs of nutrients indicate how use of limited resources can be modified to provide more people with adequate diets.

The general approach in this study is applicable to food problems in other countries although the analysis made here is confined to the United States. Not all the information necessary for detailed analysis is available, but there is enough to point to some very significant conclusions.

FOOD NEEDS FOR BETTER NUTRITION

NATIONAL CONSUMPTION TRENDS

Before turning to detailed estimates of food needs to provide better diets, it is well to consider briefly recent trends in consumption. Total food consumption per person did not change greatly from 1909 to 1939, whether measured in total pounds or with 1935–39 average prices for products (fig. 1). But there were some significant changes for individual products. Since 1909 there has been a gradual trend toward more dairy products, citrus fruit and tomatoes, and leafy, green, and yellow vegetables and less grain products and potatoes (fig. 3). Consumption of eggs, meats, and fats fluctuated from year to year, but showed no long-term trends. However, consumption of all livestock products, citrus fruits, and vegetables has increased greatly since before the last war, and this is responsible for the large increase in per capita consumption of all foods combined.

The national average diet has improved greatly in nutritional quality since 1909 and especially during the last few years (fig. 4). There has been a shift from foods relatively high in caloric content to foods relatively high in minerals and vitamins. The gradual increase in supplies of ascorbic acid and vitamin A are mainly from increased consumption of citrus fruits and vegetables, while larger supplies of calcium and riboflavin are mainly from dairy products. The very significant increase in per capita consumption of all nutrients except carbohydrates since 1939 was brought about by greatly increased consumption of foods especially high in the nutrients in which many diets were deficient. These include whole-milk products, meat and poultry, eggs, citrus fruit and tomatoes, and leafy, green, and yellow vegetables. Improvement of the nutritional quality of certain foods also has been important. For example, enrichment of flour and fortification of cereal products are responsible for a large part of the increases shown for iron, thiamine, riboflavin, and niacin since before the last war *(4, p. 20)*.

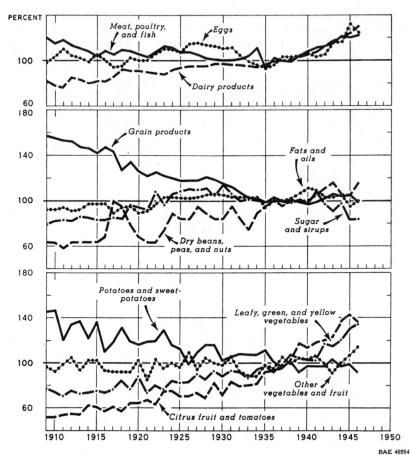

FIGURE 3.—Apparent per capita consumption of foods by major groups, United States, 1909–46.   (Index numbers 1935–39 = 100.)

FOOD-NUTRIENT NEEDS

Many people in this country do not have diets that are adequate from a nutritional standpoint despite the improvements that have resulted with higher rates of food consumption in recent years.   Per capita consumption of food nutrients and food products has been great enough, on a national average basis, to provide a relatively high average level of nutrition (tables 1 and 2).   But there are large differences in consumption between the various population groups.   This is shown by two detailed surveys of food consumption.   One was made in 1936 and the other in 1942.   It was estimated from the 1936 study

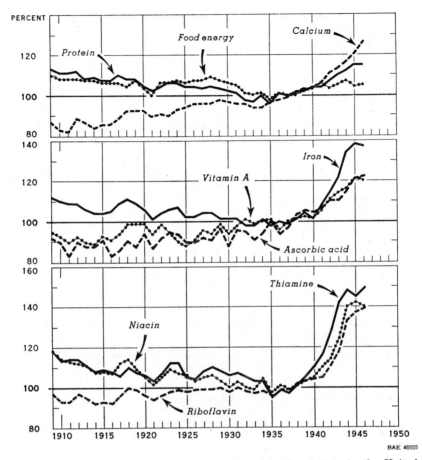

FIGURE 4.—Apparent per capita consumption of food nutrients in the United States, 1909–46. (Index numbers 1935–39=100.)

that fewer than one-fifth of all families had diets that met the National Research Council's recommendations for all of the seven nutrients considered (*34, p. 34*). Estimates made from the 1942 study indicate that one-half of all families did not have diets that met recommended allowances for riboflavin, one-third did not meet the allowances for calcium, one-fourth for thiamine, and about one-tenth for ascorbic acid, vitamin A, iron and protein (*34, pp. 34–35*). Recent findings about the nutrient content of foods and requirements for individual nutrients might modify these estimates, but it still would be true that many people do not have adequate diets (*21*).

TABLE 1.—*Apparent per capita consumption of foods by major groups, United States, averages 1935–39, 1941–45, and 1946, and adequate diet plans (retail weights)*

Food group	Average [1]			Adequate diet plans [2]	
	1935–39	1941–45	1946	Low cost	Moder- ate cost
	Pounds	*Pounds*	*Pounds*	*Pounds*	*Pounds*
Dairy products (excluding butter)[3]___	441	512	574	533	628
Eggs_____	36	41	45	33	45
Meat, poultry, game, fish_____	137	159	167	90	132
Fats and oils (including fat cuts and butter)_____	64	66	64	44	44
Dry beans, peas, nuts, and soya flour_	19	21	22	19	11
Potatoes and sweetpotatoes_____	143	141	132	173	139
Citrus fruit and tomatoes_____	84	107	114	120	146
Leafy, green, and yellow vegetables__	100	117	134	122	172
Other vegetables and fruit_____	220	221	250	95	178
Grain products_____	197	203	195	193	165
Sugar and sirups_____	109	104	92	38	45

[1] From CLARK, FRIEND, and BURK (*4*) and revised estimates for years since 1941 from THE NATIONAL FOOD SITUATION. Bur. Agr. Econ., October-December 1947, 42 pp. (Processed.)

[2] From Bureau of Human Nutrition and Home Economics (*36*). These diet plans differ slightly from prewar recommended diets. Desirable diet-plans were developed for different age, sex, and level-of-activity groups, and these were weighted by 1947 population data showing the distribution of groups among the total population, to obtain the averages shown here.

[3] Milk equivalent calculated on basis of protein and calcium content.

TABLE 2.—*Nutrients available per capita per day in the United States, averages 1935–39, 1941–45, and 1946, the recommended allowances of the National Research Council, and the nutrient content of adequate diet plans*

| Food nutrient | Unit | Average [1] | | | N. R. C. recommended allowances [2] | Adequate diet plans [3] | |
		1935–39	1941–45	1946		Low cost	Moderate cost
Food energy	Calorie	3,250	3,408	3,400	2,640	2,720	2,810
Protein	Gram	89	98	102	65	85	92
Fat	do	132	141	144			
Carbohydrate	do	428	434	420			
Calcium	Milligram	900	1,018	1,130	940	1,080	1,250
Iron	do	14	17	19	11.7	15.0	15.9
Vitamin A	International unit	8,100	9,180	9,700	4,580	8,530	10,330
Thiamine	Milligram	1.5	2.1	2.3	1.30	1.8	1.9
Riboflavin	do	1.9	2.2	2.6	1.78	2.2	2.5
Niacin	do	15	19	22	13.0	17.0	17.8
Ascorbic acid	do	115	129	140	71	128	159

[1] From CLARK, FRIEND, and BURK (4) and revised estimates for years since 1941 from THE NATIONAL FOOD SITUATION. Bur. Agr. Econ. 42 pp., October–December 1947. (Processed.) Nutrients indicated are those contained in the food brought into kitchens; they make no allowances for wastes or cooking losses.

[2] From National Research Council (20). Recommended dietary allowances for different age, sex, and level-of-activity groups weighted by distribution of population among groups in 1947, to obtain the average allowances shown here. Recommended allowances are those for nutrients actually taken into the body.

[3] From Bureau of Human Nutrition and Home Economics. Nutrients are those available in the adequate-diet plans shown in table 1. They are those contained in food brought into kitchens and make no allowance for wastes or cooking losses.

It is desirable to know approximately how much the national consumption of each food nutrient would have to be increased if the diets of those people that are below a specified level of adequacy were brought up to such a level.   The recommended dietary allowances of the National Research Council or the nutrient content of a desirable diet plan such as those developed by the Bureau of Human Nutrition and Home Economics may be used to represent such a level (table 2).

Optimal levels of consumption for most nutrients are not well established, but it is believed that for some nutrients even higher rates of consumption than those recommended by the National Research Council may have beneficial effects on health (20).

The National Research Council's recommendations are for nutrients actually taken into the body, and they must be adjusted upward to allow for normal losses in cooking and wastes in food preparation before they are directly comparable with the nutrient content of foods as brought into kitchens.   On the other hand, the diet plans developed by the Bureau of Human Nutrition and Home Economics include more of some nutrients than are required to allow for losses and wastes and to provide the National Research Council's recommended allowances (table 2).   They include foods to satisfy tastes and preferences to the extent possible with the limits set by total cost for the diet (36).[4]

There are many diet plans that will supply adequate amounts of nutrients, but because of the unequal distribution of nutrients in foods, it is difficult to devise a diet plan that will supply enough of some nutrients but not more than the recommended amounts of others.

The 1942 survey of food consumption shows average consumption of nutrients per person (contained in the food brought into kitchens) separately for urban, rural nonfarm, and rural farm families by net money income classes divided by 500-dollar intervals (34, pp. 130–131). Information is not complete enough to ascertain very accurately how much the allowances recommended by the National Research Council would have to be adjusted upward to allow for average losses and wastes in food preparation and consumption so that they would be directly comparable with these consumption data.   But it is possible to compute how much the per capita supplies of the different nutrients would have to be increased in order that average consumption within each population group might be raised to the level of the low-cost or moderate-cost diet plans.

The percentage increases that would be necessary to raise average consumption of nutrients to the level of the low-cost diet plan are as follows: Calcium 12, vitamin A 10, ascorbic acid 10, niacin 8, iron 7, thiamine 5, and riboflavin 5.[5]   Those that would be required to achieve the level of moderate-cost diet are as follows: Calcium 30, vitamin A 38, ascorbic acid 23, iron 13, niacin 12, thiamine 9, riboflavin 12, and protein 3.

---

[4] Other desirable diet plans have been developed in the past.   For example, see BUREAU OF HUMAN NUTRITION and HOME ECONOMICS.   PLANNING DIETS BY THE NEW YARDSTICK OF GOOD NUTRITION: LOW COST, MODERATE COST AND LIBERAL. 14 pp., July 1941.   (Processed.)

[5] These percentage increases in per capita supplies of nutrients were computed by comparing the nutrient content of the low-cost and moderate-cost diet plans for a moderately active man, a nutrition unit, with the average consumption of nutrients in the foods brought into kitchens per nutrition unit in the different population groups, as indicated by the 1942 survey of food consumption (34, p. 131).

As consumption of nutrients was lowest among people with low incomes, according to the 1942 survey, they would have to increase their consumption more than indicated by these average percentages. On the other hand, smaller percentage increases would be required among the high-income groups. It is significant that consumption of food energy averaged higher in all income groups than that contained in the adequate diet plans.

It should be understood that the percentage increases in per capita supplies of nutrients listed above would be sufficient only to raise *average* consumption within those population groups, whose average consumption was below the quantity of nutrients contained in the low-cost and the moderate-cost diets, to these levels (table 2). They would not be large enough to provide all people in these population groups with nutrients in the quantities contained in the adequate-diet plans if nutrients are distributed unequally among people within the groups. Furthermore, some people in other population groups whose average consumption of nutrients was as great as, or higher than, that contained in the adequate-diet plans may not have received nutrients in these quantities because of unequal distribution of consumption among people within the groups. The percentage increases in per capita supplies of nutrients listed above, of course, do not include allowances for raising the consumption of these people.

The low-cost and moderate-cost diet plans may contain more of some nutrients than necessary to provide the allowances recommended by the National Research Council, even if they were adjusted upward to allow for average losses and wastes in food preparation and consumption. Because of the unequal distribution of nutrients in foods, it is necessary to consume more of some nutrients than would be required to supply the National Research Council's recommended allowances in order to have enough of others, if they are to be made available in diets similar to those which generally are consumed.

A more adequate supply of nutrients would be made available, of course, if per capita supplies were raised so that average consumption of nutrients in all population groups could be as high as the nutrient content of the moderate-cost diet than if they were raised only enough to equal the content of the low-cost diet. But the increases that would make possible a level of nutrient consumption as high as that of the low-cost diet would be large enough to provide the recommended allowances of the National Research Council. Therefore they may be considered minimum desirable increases in 1942 per capita supplies of nutrients. Per capita supplies of nutrients have averaged somewhat higher in the last few years than they did in 1942 (fig. 4). As a result, these increases from recent wartime supplies of nutrients per capita would make possible the achievement of adequate diets for all. This would be true even if there were some unequal distribution of nutrients within population groups.

FOOD-PRODUCT NEEDS

National consumption of food products could be changed in many ways to supply the increases in food nutrients indicated above as necessary, if all diets below a specified level of adequacy were to be brought up to such a level. It would be possible, for example, to increase the total supply of nutrients by these quantities, without employing more resources to expand food production, by changing the national pattern of production and consumption to include more of the products that provide large outputs of nutrients per unit of resources in place of those that provide small outputs. But, this would involve shifts in consumption of foods which consumers would not like to make and which would not be necessary if the additional nutrients can be made available by increasing the total supply of food products.

If all people had diets similar to those developed by the Bureau of Human Nutrition and Home Economics (table 1), they of course would receive adequate quantities of the different nutrients. The 1942 survey of food consumption shows the average quantities of the various foods consumed per person separately for urban, rural non-farm, and rural farm groups by net money income classes, divided by 500-dollar intervals (34, p. 7). Therefore it is possible to compute how much per capita consumption of the different foods would have to be increased if all groups whose average consumption was below the adequate diet plans were to be raised to these levels. The percentage increases that would be required to provide the low-cost diet are as follows: Milk or its equivalent 19; green, leafy, and yellow vegetables 12; tomatoes and citrus fruit 10; meat, poultry, and fish 3; grain products 13; potatoes and sweetpotatoes 19; and dry beans and peas 17. The percentage increases that would be necessary to provide the moderate-cost diet are: Milk or its equivalent 36; green, leafy, and yellow vegetables 31; tomatoes and citrus fruit 30; other vegetables and fruit 14; meat, poultry, and fish 18; eggs 1; grain products 3; and potatoes and sweetpotatoes 2. Per capita consumption of many of these products has been upward since 1942 (fig. 3, p. 6).

These changes in per capita consumption would provide the additional quantities of nutrients that were estimated as necessary if average consumption of nutrients within the different population groups that were below the nutrient content of either the low-cost or moderate-cost plans were to be raised to these levels. Of course it would be necessary that the additional products be distributed according to needs, if all diets were to be raised to these levels. Total food consumption per capita would be about 8 percent higher if measured in value terms, and 11 percent higher if measured in total pounds, than it was in 1942 if the increases required to provide the low-cost diet plan were achieved. It would be about 18 percent higher if measured in value terms and 20 percent higher if measured in total pounds, if the increases required to achieve the moderate-cost diet were achieved.

Both sets of consumption changes probably would be possible from a physical standpoint because they would involve less than a 10-percent increase in consumption of food energy. Increases in consumption of food energy are not needed from a nutritional standpoint, and it is probable that consumption of foods that have a high content of food energy in relation to other nutrients such as cereals and potatoes would be reduced if more of the highly nutritious foods were consumed.

Estimates of the national increases in consumption of food products which would improve diets were also made in a recent study by

Cochrane (5).   Per capita consumption data for farm and nonfarm families and single persons, by net money income groups by 500-dollar intervals, were available from the 1936 survey.   These consumption data were extrapolated forward in accordance with changes in domestic disappearance of food products from 1936 to 1941.[6]   A diet plan drawn up by the Bureau of Human Nutrition and Home Economics then was compared with actual consumption of food products to learn how much consumption would have to be increased in those groups below the diet level to raise them to this level.[7]   It was assumed that those groups whose average consumption was equal to or above the diet plan for any food group would continue to consume this much.

The percentage increases in per capita consumption from the 1941 actual consumption were estimated as follows: Milk or its equivalent 46; eggs 6; meat, poultry, and fish 5; potatoes and sweetpotatoes 4; tomatoes and citrus fruit 24; leafy green and yellow vegetables 79; and other vegetables and fruit 4.   The additional products are relatively high in minerals and vitamins in relation to caloric content. These increases in per capita consumption of food products would provide more than enough of each nutrient to make possible the increases estimated above as necessary to raise average consumption of nutrients within each population group to the level of the moderate-cost diet plan (table 2).   Total food consumption per capita would be about 15 percent higher when measured in value terms, and 20 percent higher when measured in total pounds than in 1941, if these changes in consumption were accomplished.   There are of course many other ways in which consumption of food products could be changed to supply the same increases in supplies of nutrients if total food supplies per capita could be increased 15 percent.

Earlier estimates of the increases in consumption of food products that would be required to provide better nutrition were made by Stiebeling after studying the results of the 1936 survey (30, p. 380). The increases in consumption necessary to have "freely chosen diets that can be rated good nutritionally" were estimated roughly as follows: Milk 20 percent, tomatoes and citrus fruit 70 percent, and leafy green, and yellow vegetables 100 percent.   These increases were described as far from optimal, and a doubling milk consumption was considered desirable from a nutritional standpoint.

The Food and Agriculture Organization of the United Nations recently set up consumption targets for most countries of the world (8).   These are in terms of increases in prewar food supplies to be required by 1950.   The targets for the United States would involve changes in consumption of food products about the same as those indicated by the estimates from Cochrane, listed above.

---

[6] See COCHRANE (5, p. 8 footnote 8) for statement of how these consumption data for 1941 were derived from the 1935–36 consumer-purchases study.   COCHRANE (5, p. 6, table 1) shows the diet that was compared with actual consumption by each income and population group to learn the extent to which national consumption must be increased to reach the "high-level" diet.

[7] The diet plan used was the moderate-cost diet described in PLANNING DIETS BY THE NEW YARDSTICK OF GOOD NUTRITION: LOW COST, MODERATE COST, AND LIBERAL.   Bur. Human Nutrition and Home Economics, 14 pp. 1941.   (Processed.)

CHANGES IN FOOD PRODUCTION

Total food production averaged about one-third higher in the 1942–45 war years than it did in the 1935–39 period if measured by valuing products at their average 1935–39 prices (fig. 5). But the total food supply made available for consumption from United States production, measured in nutritive terms, increased about one-half. Each dollar's worth of food made available for consumption in 1942–45, when valued at 1935–39 prices, contained about 15 percent more nutrients than did that made available in 1935–39. This is apparent from the fact that per capita consumption of all nutrients by civilians averaged almost 25 percent higher during the recent war years than it did just before the war although food consumption per capita (measured by 1935–39 prices for products) increased only 10 percent (figs.

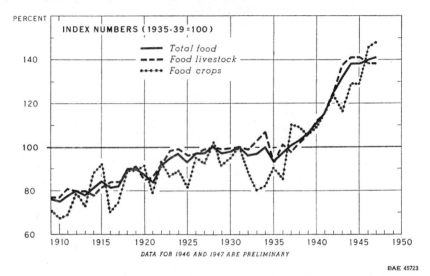

FIGURE 5.—Volume of agricultual production for sale and farm home consumption: total food, food livestock, and food crops, United States, 1909–47.

1 and 4). Of course, a large part of the total food supply was used for noncivilian purposes during the war. But the nutrient content of this part of the food supply probably increased about as much as did that consumed by civilians. The increases in supplies of nutrients were much greater for minerals and vitamins than for protein, carbohydrates, or fats.

Patriotic appeals for more food, together with a gradual doubling of prices paid for farm products, provided incentives to increase production. But these large increases would not have been possible if it had not been for several other favorable factors. Better than average weather is frequently mentioned as one cause, but careful study of weather and yield data shows that only about one-fourth of the wartime expansion in farm output can be attributed to weather. Some of the increase in livestock production was made possible by accumulated reserves of domestic wheat and feed grains, but these reserves accounted for less than 10 percent of the concentrates fed to livestock in 1944, and most of the increase in livestock products came from current feed production.[8]

In order to explain how the increased food output was achieved, it is necessary to examine in greater detail the methods of increasing the total food supply. Food production can be increased in three ways: (1) By employing more resources (land, labor, and capital goods) to produce food, (2) by using improved production techniques to obtain higher rates of output per unit of resources, and (3) by shifting the use of resources to produce more of the products that provide relatively large outputs of nutrients per unit of resources in the place of those that give small outputs. In addition, more food can be made available for consumption from fixed supplies (1) by more complete utilization of the food value contained in farm products and (2) by improving the nutritional quality of the foods produced. How much of the wartime increase in food supplies can be attributed to each of these methods?

In considering how the increases in production were achieved, it is necessary to examine the changes in the total volume of agricultural production of which food products are a major part. The measure of food production to which reference has been made includes food products produced for sale and for farm-home consumption and is a part of the total volume of agricultural production for sale and farm-home consumption. Two other measures of agricultural production have been developed recently.[9] One is farm output for human use, which is similar to the measure of total agricultural production for sale and farm-home consumption but differs substantially in some years because it includes the farm production of the current year, although some of the output may be sold in later years. The other is gross farm production, which includes farm-produced power of horses and mules as an item in farm production and in this way differs from farm output (table 3).

CHANGES IN RESOURCES EMPLOYED

The total acreage of cropland has not changed much since 1920. The acreage of crops actually harvested, however, has been about 3 percent higher during the recent war years than it was before the war. There was a small shift from nonfood to food crops. The main item here, cotton, was reduced almost 20 percent, but this provided only about 1 percent more land for other crops. Approximately 55 million acres have been released from the production of feed for horses and mules during the last 30-year period (6). This long-term trend was continued during the war and the shift to mechanized power has released about 5 million acres for food production since the immediate prewar period. This is equivalent to a little more than 1 percent of all cropland. Altogether, the cropland used for food products increased about 5 percent.

[8] *See* pp. 3–5 of JOHNSON, SHERMAN E. CHANGES IN FARMING. Bur. Agr. Econ. F. M. 58, revised 107, pp., illus. 1948. (Processed.)
[9] BARTON, GLEN T., and COOPER, MARTIN R. FARM PRODUCTION IN WAR AND PEACE. Bur. Agr. Econ. F. M. 53, 85 pp., illus. 1945. (Processed.)

Despite the decline in number of horses and mules, the total volume of power and machinery, including work animals used on farms, was about one-fourth higher during the war years than just before the war (table 3). Most types of equipment were not available in the quantities wanted by farmers, but the labor-saving types of machines most needed to carry out the food-production program were made available, and the machines on hand were used more intensively. The number of animal units of breeding stock (excluding horses) was about one-fifth higher during the war than before. This increase was made possible in part by the decline in horses and mules, but more important was the increase in total feed production.

Employment of workers on farms averaged 10 percent less in 1945 than in 1935–39, but farm people worked more hours. The farm-work load did not increase by the same percentage as total farm production because of the increased efficiency in the use of labor. The total number of man-hours of labor actually employed in all farm production was only slightly higher during the war years than immediately before, and the number of hours each person worked probably increased nearly 10 percent. Labor requirements were distributed more evenly throughout the year.[10]

TABLE 3.—*Volume of agricultural production, resources employed in agricultural production, and productivity of resources, United States, averages 1910–45 (Index numbers, 1935–39=100)* [1]

Item	Averages			
	1910–14	1915–19	1920–24	1925–29
Volume of agricultural production measures:				
Food production for sale and farm home consumption	78	86	91	97
Farm output for human use [2]	80	83	88	96
Gross farm production [2]	89	94	97	101
Resources employed in agricultural production:				
Total cropland [3]	90	96	98	100
Animal units of breeding stock [4]			105	101
Volume of all power and machinery [5]	100	107	118	114
Farm employment [6]	110	107	104	104
Total volume of all resource inputs [7]	95	99	105	106
Productivity of agricultural resources:				
Crop production per acre [8]			98	101
Livestock production per unit of livestock [9]			85	95
Farm output per unit of all power and machinery [10]	80	78	75	84
Gross production per farm worker [11]	81	88	93	97
Farm output per unit of all resource inputs [12]	84	84	84	91

See footnotes at end of table.

[10] *See* HECHT, REUBEN W. FARM LABOR REQUIREMENTS IN THE UNITED STATES, 1939 and 1944. Bur. Agr. Econ. F. M. 59, 68 pp., illus. 1947. (Processed.)

TABLE 3.—*Volume of agricultural production, resources employed in agricultural production, and productivity of resources, United States, averages 1910–45 (Index numbers, 1935–39=100)*[1]—Continued

Item	Averages			
	1930–34	1935–39	1940–44	1943–45
Volume of agricultural production measures:				
Food production for sale and farm home consumption	98	100	125	136
Farm output for human use [2]	94	100	101	128
Gross farm production [2]	96	100	117	122
Resources employed in agricultural production:				
Total cropland [3]	102	100	99	100
Animal units of breeding stock [4]	107	100	118	129
Volume of all power and machinery [5]	108	100	115	123
Farm employment [6]	101	100	95	92
Total volume of all resource inputs [7]	103	100	108	113
Productivity of agricultural resources:				
Crop production per acre [8]	92	100	117	120
Livestock production per unit of livestock [9]	95	100	108	108
Farm output per unit of all power and machinery [10]	87	100	105	104
Gross production per farm worker [11]	95	100	123	133
Farm output per unit of all resource inputs [12]	92	100	112	113

[1] All data except volume of food production for sale and farm home consumption are from COOPER, BARTON, and BRODELL (6).

[2] Farm output is gross farm production minus farm-produced power of horses and mules and measures calendar-year production of farm products for human use. Gross farm production measures calendar-year production of all crops and pasture consumed by all livestock, and the product added in the conversion of feed and pasture into livestock and livestock products for human use and the farm-produced power of horses and mules. *See* BARTON, GLEN T., and COOPER, MARTIN R. FARM PRODUCTION IN WAR AND PEACE. Bur. Agr. Econ. F. M. 53, 85 pp., illus. 1945. (Processed.)

[3] Total cropland is the sum of estimated acreage of land from which one or more crops were harvested, plus estimated crop failure and summer-fallow acreage.

[4] Combined volume calculated by weighting annual numbers of livestock (except horses and mules) and poultry on farms by their 1935–39 average contribution to livestock production.

[5] Combined volume calculated by weighting annual numbers of motor vehicles, machines, equipment, and horses and mules on farms by their 1935–39 average values.

[6] Average annual farm employment as reported by Bureau of Agricultural Economics.

[7] Combined volume of all resource inputs including land, labor, livestock, machines, and supplies by weighting annual quantities by their 1935–39 average prices.

[8] Computed by dividing total volume of all cropland production by total acres of cropland.

[9] Computed by dividing combined volume of all livestock production for human use by number of animal units of breeding livestock.

[10] Computed by dividing farm output for human use by volume of all power and machinery.

[11] Computed by dividing gross farm production by farm employment.

[12] Computed by dividing farm output for human use by total volume of all resource inputs in agriculture.

It is possible to combine all the resource inputs used in agricultural production into a single measure of resource input by valuing them at their cost rates in the 1935–39 period (table 3). The total volume of all resource inputs in agricultural production was 13 percent higher in 1943–45 than in 1935–39, according to this measure. Factors that account for this are the increased volume of power and machinery and the increased volume of other supplies such as lime and fertilizer.

Effects of Improved Production Techniques

Approximately one-half of the wartime expansion in agricultural production can be attributed to increased employment of resources and one-half to higher rates of output per unit of resources. With no change in the efficiency with which resources are used, a 13-percent increase in the total volume of resource inputs of course would have caused total farm output to be increased 13 percent. But farm output per unit of all resource inputs also increased 13 percent.

Crop production per acre was about 20 percent higher and livestock production per animal unit of breeding stock was nearly 10 percent higher during the war years than before the war. Gross farm production per worker increased about one-third, but a part of this was the result of more hours of work. Farm output per unit of all power and machinery including work animals did not increase greatly, but these resources were used in larger quantities and helped to make possible higher rates of output per acre and per farm worker.

These increases in productivity were made possible by technological improvements that have gradually become available through scientific research and were rapidly put into effect when war called for virtually all-out food production. They include higher yielding varieties of crops, better feeding and improved breeds of livestock, greater use of fertilizer and lime, increased use of cover crops and conservation practices, and better control of pests and disease. Among improved crop varieties, the wide adoption of hybrid corn (which generally has a yield 20 percent higher than the open-pollinated varieties) and higher yielding varieties of oats and soybeans were most important.[11] Livestock rations were better balanced by the increased use of protein supplements made available from the expansion in vegetable-oil crops and by more digestible protein from the larger production of legume hay. Total supplies of protein oil meals have increased about one-half since before the war. Among the oil crops, increased production of soybeans, which expanded about four times, was most important. The long-term trend toward more legume hay, which has increased the digestible protein in all hay about one-third since 1920, was continued.[12] Fertilizer consumption doubled during the war and helped to make possible higher crop yields.[13] In addition, the longer term effects of lime application in connection with soil conservation and improvement programs showed up forcefully.

[11] Crickman, C. W. feed grains and meat animals in war and peace. Bur. Agr. Econ. F. M. 51, 55 pp., illus. 1945. (Processed) and Strand, E. G. soybrean production in war and peace. Bur. Agr. Econ. F. M. 50, 41 pp., illus. 1945. (Processed.)
[12] Johnson, N. W. changes in hay production in war and peace. Bur. Agr. Econ. F. M. 47, 37 pp. illus. 1945. (Processed.)
[13] Ibach, D. B. cropland use and soil fertility practice in war and peace. Bur. Agr. Econ. F. M. 52, 58 pp. illus. 1946. (Processed.)

The large farm production in recent years was made possible without employing additional labor by greater use of the more efficient production techniques. Improved mechanical methods, which have replaced horse and mule power as well as much hand labor, helped to get farm jobs done on time—especially planting, cultivating, and harvesting. Greater use of tractors, combines, milking machines, and other farm implements has come gradually, but the wartime demand for food gave an additional push to this development. Of course, higher yields per acre and increased efficiency of livestock in the use of feed also helped to raise the productivity of farm workers.

The improved techniques that have brought about increased efficiency in agricultural production undoubtedly will continue to be used because most of them will be profitable regardless of changes in demand for farm products. For example, better yielding varieties of crops and more efficient livestock do not require much, if any, additional cash outlay and are likely to be profitable even though farm prices may decline. A large part of the increased agricultural production has been achieved by the use of more resource inputs, and most of them will continue to be used regardless of changes in conditions of demand. The volume of power and machinery and the number of animal units of breeding stock have increased greatly, and cash costs of farm production cannot be reduced very much by discontinuing their use. The same applies to land and labor, which together constitute the bulk of resource inputs used in agriculture. Annual expenditures for such items as fertilizer and lime now are much higher than formerly, but many farmers will find their use profitable on the present expanded scale even though farm prices decline.

Therefore it is not probable that the total volume of resource inputs will decline greatly. Instead, they probably will increase, as required to bring about increased efficiency or expansion in production. Total agricultural production will continue to increase as scientific research makes improved production methods possible, although the rate at which they are put into effect will depend upon their profitableness, and this in turn will depend largely upon conditions of demand.

EFFECTS OF PRODUCTION SHIFTS

Food production was increased about 3 percent more than the total volume of agricultural production between the 1935–39 and 1943–45 periods. Total output of nonfood products averaged slightly lower, and all of the net increase in agricultural production was in food products. This means that a larger proportion of the available farm resources have been used to produce food in the years just past.

Production was expanded much more for certain items than for others, to meet special war needs (fig. 6). There was no pronounced tendency, however, to produce more of the products that have a relatively high output of nutrients from the resources used, in place of those that have a low output, although changes generally were in this direction. The adjustments were toward an over-all expansion in food production with emphasis on those products that could be expanded most quickly and at the same time would meet particular food needs.

Record stocks of grain were on hand at the beginning of the war when demand for livestock products shot upward. The immediate

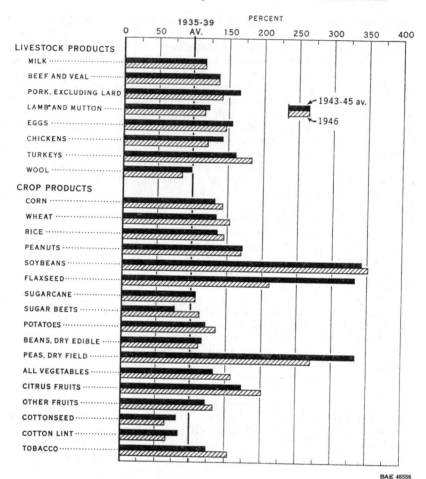

FIGURE 6.—Production of selected farm products, 1943–45 average and 1946 as percentages of 1935–39 average, United States.

objective, therefore, was to get grains converted into livestock products as rapidly as possible. The production of hogs and eggs could be expanded more quickly than dairying, and so they increased most. Farmers were encouraged to expand feed crops in order to maintain a high level of livestock production. But by the end of the war, feed reserves had mostly disappeared, although the ratio of grain prices to livestock prices continued to favor feeding. By this time the need of food to prevent starvation in foreign countries was growing rapidly. Cereals, which are especially economical as sources of energy and certain minerals and vitamins, were demanded most, so farmers were asked to market their cereals, especially wheat, directly rather than in the form of livestock products.

Supplies of fats and oils usually imported from the Pacific Islands were cut off early in the war.[14] To make up these losses, the produc-

[14] HANSEN, P. L. WORLD TRENDS IN MAJOR OIL CROPS. Bur. Agr. Econ. F. M. 54, 62 pp., illus. 1946. (Processed.)

tion of peanuts, soybeans, and flaxseed was greatly expanded. Other significant changes among the food crops were increases in potatoes, dry beans and peas, rice, citrus fruit, and certain vegetables that could be canned. All these are products that have a relatively high output of nutrients per unit of resources used in production. Among the major crops only cotton was reduced, and almost enough cotton for a year's consumption had been carried over from one year to the next for several years.

The pattern of food production had changed enough by the end of the war to make possible significant changes in consumption, and they greatly improved the nutritive value of the national diet. Per capita consumption of citrus fruit, certain vegetables, meat, eggs, and dairy products, excluding butter, was increased; only in the case of sugar and fats did consumption decline. Per capita consumption of food energy was increased about 5 percent, although supplies of sugar and fats, which are the source of about one-third of the food energy in the diet, decreased about 10 percent. Increased consumption of livestock products and fruits and vegetables more than made up the loss of energy from these sources and at the same time made possible much higher consumption rates for protein, minerals, and vitamins. The greater importance of livestock products (excluding butter, lard, and fat cuts of meat) in the national diet is illustrated by the fact that in the prewar period of 1935–39 they were the source of 24 percent of the calories and 54 percent of the protein, while in the 1944–45 period they accounted for 27 percent of the calories and 58 percent of the protein (4, p. 22).

Changes in the pattern of food production do not account for the larger volume of food output measured in monetary terms, but they are an important source of increased food supplies measured in terms of food nutrients. As has been explained, food production measured in nutritive items increased about 15 percent more than did food production measured by products valued at 1935–39 average prices. Approximately one-third of this 15-percent increase can be attributed to changes in the pattern of production and two-thirds to more complete utilization of the nutritive content of foods.

BETTER UTILIZATION OF FOOD SUPPLIES

Among the changes in the utilization of food supplies during the war, the increased use of nonfat solids in milk was most important. Per capita consumption of nonfat solids was 25 percent higher in 1945 than before the war although total milk production increased only 16 percent. The proportion of all nonfat solids in the milk supply used for human consumption was raised from 55 percent in the prewar period to approximately 70 percent in 1945. As all of the nonfat solids in the milk produced are not even now being used for human consumption, this still is a noteworthy potential source of additional food. Additional facilities for processing and distribution would be necessary if these products are to be made available to consumers.

How much could per capita consumption of individual nutrients be increased by complete utilization of all the solids in milk now being produced? Nonfat milk solids was the source of 24 percent of the protein, 74 percent of the calcium, and 45 percent of the riboflavin in the national diet, in 1944–45. Complete utilization of the nonfat solids of milk could be the source of approximately 5 percent more protein, 30 percent more calcium, and 10 percent more riboflavin. This does not necessarily mean that a greater production of milk, especially in certain areas, would not be a more efficient source of

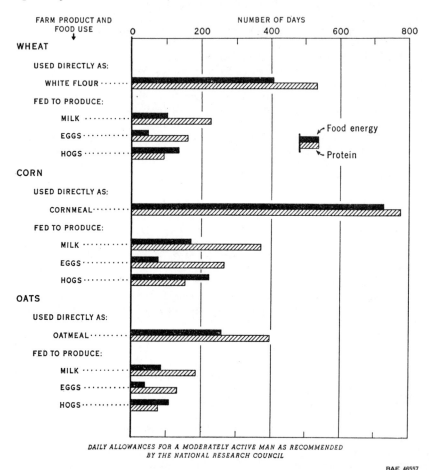

DAILY ALLOWANCES FOR A MODERATELY ACTIVE MAN AS RECOMMENDED
BY THE NATIONAL RESEARCH COUNCIL

BAE 46557

FIGURE 7.—Number of days a man could be supplied with a daily allowance of food energy and protein by an acre of land used to produce selected products, United States (1941–45 average yields).

these nutrients than complete utilization of milk in areas where it is now being produced.

Diversion of cereals from livestock to human consumption could be an important source of additional food supplies. Wheat provides 5 to 10 times as many calories when consumed directly as when converted into livestock products and eaten as meat, lard, butter, or milk (fig. 7). Plentiful supplies of energy foods made unnecessary any very substantial shifts from livestock to crop products during the war. Consumption of grain products has averaged only 3 percent higher in recent years than before the war despite the reduction in supplies of other highly concentrated energy foods, such as sugar and fats. Slightly more peanuts and soybeans were consumed in whole form, but most of the protein from the increased production was used as livestock feed, and only the oil was used directly as human food.

Some of the food nutrients that would be required in larger quantities to provide better nutrition could be supplied by diversion of cereals and other crop products to human consumption. But because of their bulk and high caloric content, relative to mineral and vitamin content, consumption of these products cannot be increased enough to meet a very large part of nutritional shortages. An increase in consumption of grain products results in approximately the same percentage increase in food energy as in iron, thiamine, niacin, and riboflavin, which are the most plentiful nutrients in grain products. For example, a 20-percent increase in consumption of grain products would result in about 5 percent more calories and at the same time only 5 percent more iron, thiamine, and niacin.

More food, especially minerals and vitamins, could be obtained from a fixed supply of grain by increasing the rates of flour extraction. Milling ratios were not increased during the war, but early in 1946 they were temporarily raised from about 70 to 80 percent in order to conserve wheat, which had become short in supply relative to needs, especially for foreign-relief purposes. If whole-grain products rather than refined products were consumed, per capita consumption of the important nutrients contained in grain such as protein, calcium, iron, thiamine, niacin, and riboflavin would be increased greatly. But because of consumer preferences for refined products, it is exceedingly difficult to increase the consumption of the nutrients that are deficient in diets very much by this method. Even in foreign countries, where rates of flour extraction are much higher than in the United States, whole-grain products are not eaten in very large quantities.

An outstanding development during the war which greatly improved the nutritional quality of grain products is the enrichment of flour and fortification of breakfast cereals. The percentage increases in per capita consumption of nutrients resulting from enrichment have been estimated as follows: iron 17, thiamine 27, niacin 19, and riboflavin 13 (4, p. 20). Enrichment of flour has not met with the full approval of all nutrition authorities, but the addition of dried skim milk in the preparation of baking products is widely recognized as desirable.

Prevention of food waste is another method of obtaining more food from fixed supplies. It has been estimated that nearly one-fourth of the food produced in the United States is not utilized (14). Much of this loss is unavoidable, but the waste can be reduced considerably. Food wastes occur on farms because of incomplete harvesting at times when market prices are relatively low; some occur in marketing because of the inadequacy of refrigeration and other facilities. As to the losses in preparation of foods in homes and restaurants, Raymond Pearl, chief statistician of the Food Administration in the first World War, estimated wastage of food in the homes to be 5 percent of the protein, 25 percent of the fats, 20 percent of the carbohydrates, and 19 percent of the total calories (23). Measures to prevent wastes caused by failure to harvest all the crops completely (especially fruits and vegetables), and by inadequate marketing facilities must be balanced against additional costs. But waste of edible food in homes and restaurants can be avoided with little or no additional expense.

IMPROVING THE NUTRITIONAL QUALITY OF FOODS

Closely related to better utilization of available food supplies is improvement in the nutritional quality of food produced. A food may vary in nutritional value as a result of conditions under which it is produced. These include mineral content of soils, climatic conditions, and varieties of plants. L. A. Maynard, an authority on this subject, says:

> Tomatoes, upon which we rely for vitamin C, may range from 5 to 45 mg. of the vitamin in the fresh fruit. Butter may range from 5,000 to 25,000 I. U. of vitamin A per pound. Such wide variations may be interpreted by some to mean that little dependence can be placed on vitamin values actually obtained from these sources. But this is the wrong interpretation, for the bulk of products as marketed exhibit much narrower ranges, and supplies from different sources eaten by the individual over any extended period tend to average up. The much more important significance of these wide ranges lies in the possibilities thus indicated of producing more of the products having the higher values, and thus of stepping up the average content of the general supply through an understanding and control of factors responsible for variations (16, pp. 7–8).

Much of the research on the physical problems of farm production has been concerned with increasing crop yields. Relatively little attention has been given to the nutritive value of the food produced. The effects of soil conditions on crop yields were recognized early, so considerable information is available about the relationships between the mineral composition of soils and the plants grown in them (2). A number of investigations in recent years concern the vitamin contents of different crop varieties. An outstanding example is an investigation of the vitamin C content of apples, reported by Maynard (15, p. 11). A variety new to the United States, the Nelson apple from New Zealand, is reported to have a vitamin C content greater than tomatoes and almost as high as citrus fruits. As most varieties of apples have a relatively low content of this nutrient, the introduction of such a new variety might eventually have a positive influence in improving diets.

Not enough is known about the effects of plant varieties, soil, and climatic conditions on the nutritive value of food products to make possible any rapid progress in improving the nutritional content of the food supply by controlling these conditions, but it is apparent that the possibilities are great. Even though gains made in this way are small and not spectacular, they are definite and may be enduring, and they can reach all groups of the population. Furthermore, it is a method of improving diets generally that demands little or no additional production resources.

RELATIVE EFFICIENCY OF PRODUCTS AS SOURCES OF FOOD NUTRIENTS

The relative efficiency of products as sources of food nutrients can be estimated by comparing the output of food nutrients per unit of resources used to produce each product. The most significant relationships are those that apply to marginal changes in the national production of individual products, but average relationships may be considered a first step in this direction. It is especially desirable to know how the output of food nutrients differs when the same resources are used to produce different products. Outputs of food nutrients per acre of land, per unit of feed in the case of livestock products, per day of farm labor, per unit of all farm resources, and per unit of all farm and nonfarm resources used to make food products available at retail, are measured in the analysis that follows. This information makes it possible to estimate the proportions of all resources used to produce particular food products or groups of products. It also provides a basis for deciding how many people could be supported with different diets, from the available resources.

Food Production per Acre of Land

The output of food per acre used to produce each product can be measured, although it must be recognized that farm land differs greatly in quality. The number of days a moderately active man can be supplied with a daily allowance of different food nutrients by an acre of land used to produce selected products in the 1941–45 period is shown in table 4. More detailed data for a longer list of products are shown in tables 20, 21, 22, and 23. The daily allowances are those recommended by the National Research Council (20).[15] The number of days' supply of five vitamins (which include vitamin A, ascorbic acid, thiamine, niacin, and riboflavin) were combined into a single measure of output by averaging the number of days computed separately for each vitamin. The number of days' supply of 10 nutrients (which include food energy, protein, fat, calcium, and iron, in addition to the 5 vitamins) were combined by averaging the days computed separately for each nutrient. This procedure has the effect of giving equal weight to each nutrient in the proportions recommended by the National Research Council. This method provides a measure of total output that is not altogether arbitrary, although it does not take into account the higher economic values that may be placed on some nutrients than on others because they are relatively scarce in the total food supply.

In making comparisons between products, it is necessary to consider the quantities in which they are usually eaten. It would not be possible to consume any one product in large enough quantities to supply daily allowances of all the nutrients. In fact, many products could not be consumed in large enough quantities to supply daily allowances of any one nutrient. For example, fruits and vegetables have large outputs of nutrients per acre of land, but they are not important sources of food energy, protein, or fat (table 11, p. 40).

The quantities of nutrients obtained from each farm product are affected by the way the product is used; therefore the manner of use is indicated. Losses in weight that occur in converting farm products into food at retail are taken into account by the application of average conversion factors.[16] The nutrient content of the food made available at retail was determined from average composition data (35). No

---

[15] See footnote 1 of table 4 for a list of these allowances.

[16] These are the same as those used by the Bureau of Agricultural Economics, in computing price spreads between farm products and food at retail (31) and shown in UNITED STATES WAR FOOD ADMINISTRATION, OFFICE OF DISTRIBUTION. CONVERSION FACTORS AND WEIGHTS AND MEASURES FOR AGRICULTURAL COMMODITIES AND THEIR PRODUCTS. 87 pp. 1944. Washington, D. C. (Processed.)

allowance is made for loss in nutritive content of food after it leaves the retail stores or for waste in home preparation. Furthermore, the output data do not include the food that is obtained indirectly from byproducts, such as bran from wheat or pulp from sugar beets, if they are fed to livestock. The importance of these byproducts and others that are sources of nonfood products is indicated by the percentage that their imputed farm value is of the total value of the farm product. These percentages are indicated in the more detailed tables, but adjustments in output data to make allowance for byproducts or joint products would not greatly affect the comparisons.

TABLE 4.—*Average outputs of food nutrients per acre of land used to produce specified products in terms of the number of days a moderately active man can be supplied with a daily allowance (1941–45 average yields)* [1]

Farm product and food use	Food energy	Protein	Fat	Calcium	5 vitamins [2]	10 nutrients [3]
	Days	*Days*	*Days*	*Days*	*Days*	*Days*
Livestock products:						
Milk, whole	108	236	245	696	157	210
Eggs	54	188	158	70	98	119
Chickens	40	180	105	12	73	80
Hogs	183	129	765	7	228	236
Cattle, all	27	77	88	4	47	50
Field crops:						
Wheat, white flour	405	527	41	81	77	163
Corn, cornmeal	725	773	294	136	740	697
Potatoes	806	812	43	391	2, 247	1, 496
Sugar beets, sugar	2, 199	0	0	0	0	234
Beans, dry edible	414	1, 116	71	656	483	773
Peanuts, peanut butter	355	643	1, 099	160	445	475
Vegetables, fresh:						
Beets	442	661	34	985	1, 235	1, 072
Cabbage	373	773	110	2, 235	6, 303	3, 667
Carrots	878	1, 009	235	2, 869	30, 500	16, 141
Lettuce	165	471	70	748	1, 620	1, 071
Onions	769	951	133	1, 900	1, 639	1, 389
Peas, green	170	486	27	140	964	645
Sweet corn	187	274	84	60	518	342
Tomatoes	141	266	74	255	2, 346	1, 340
Fruit, fresh:						
Apples	401	80	100	140	484	361
Oranges	769	582	131	1, 898	7, 154	4, 067
Plums	402	214	60	455	1, 210	809
Strawberries	120	101	70	308	1, 552	895

[1] Daily allowances are those recommended by the National Research Council for a moderately active man and are as follows: Food energy—3,000 calories, protein—70 grams, calcium—800 milligrams, iron—12 milligrams, vitamin A—5,000 International Units, thiamine—1.5 milligrams, riboflavin—2.0 milligrams, niacin—15 milligrams, and ascorbic acid—75 milligrams. No recommended allowance is given for fat, but it is considered desirable that 20 to 25 percent of the food energy be in this form. This is the basis for the recommendation of 67 grams used here. See tables 20, 21, 22, and 23, for additional data about these and other products (*20*).

[2] A simple average of the number of days computed separately for vitamin A, ascorbic acid, thiamine, riboflavin, and niacin.

[3] A simple average of the number of days computed separately for food energy, protein, fat, calcium, iron, and the 5 vitamins.

In interpreting the comparisons made in table 4 (and later in tables 20, 21, 22, and 23), the differences in the average quality of the land used to produce different products should be considered. Vegetables generally provide the most nutrients per acre, but they usually are grown on the most productive land and are fertilized most heavily. The food obtained from hogs and poultry which consume grain feeds can be compared directly with the food obtained from corn, oats, and barley when they are used as human food in the form of corn meal, oat meal, or pearl barley. On the other hand, much of the land used to support the roughage-consuming livestock—cattle and sheep—is relatively low in natural productivity. The figures for the average crop yields in the United States of the feeds actually fed to produce each livestock product were used to estimate the acreage requirements.[17] Feed from pasture was converted to a cropland-equivalent basis by computing the acreage of tame hay that would be required to provide a quantity of feed equivalent to that provided by pasture.

Some significant differences among products are apparent, even after allowance is made for differences in the quality of land used to produce different foods. For example, several food crops provide 5 to 10 times as much food energy as do hogs—the most efficient source among livestock. Land used to produce milk for use in whole-milk products provides about one-half as much protein, calcium, and ribo-flavin as do the most efficient sources among food crops, although they provide considerably more than do many others. Other food nutrients, including iron, vitamin A, ascorbic acid, thiamine, and niacin, can be obtained most efficiently from field crops, vegetables, and fruits.

In general, the land suitable for crop production will produce most if it is devoted to food crops for direct human consumption, whereas the land suitable only for growing roughage feeds will be most productive if used to produce milk for use in whole form. But great shifts in land use such as these are not necessary to the meeting of food requirements.

FOOD FROM FEED

Livestock provide about one-third of all the food energy contained in the national diet, but they consume about three times as much food energy as do all people in the United States. Therefore only about one-ninth of the calories consumed by livestock are made available for human consumption. But livestock perform a valuable service in transforming roughage feeds that are unsuitable for human use into foods that are highly concentrated in protein, minerals, and vitamins, in relation to calories. About two-thirds of the feed fed to livestock consists of roughage feeds. In addition, part of the grains is in the form of inedible concentrates.

As about 80 percent of all the farm land used to produce the national food supply is devoted to livestock production, it is especially important during periods of food shortages to know how livestock products compare in efficiency as sources of food nutrients from feed (17). The numbers of days that a moderately active man can be supplied with a daily allowance of each of the food nutrients from 1,000 units of feed used to produce different livestock products are shown in table 5 (and

---

[17] Data on feed consumption on which the estimates are based are from JEN-NINGS, R. D. FEED CONSUMED BY LIVESTOCK, 1941–42, BY STATES. Bur. Agr. Econ. 108 pp., illus. 1946. (Processed.)

later in table 24).   A feed unit is defined as 1 pound of corn or equivalent quantities of other feeds.   For example, a feed unit roughly equals 2 pounds of hay or 5 pounds of corn silage.   The rates for converting feeds to a unit basis depend upon their content of total digestible nutrients and protein.   Feed requirements for producing the different livestock products are national average data.

Milk used in whole form is the most efficient source of protein, calcium, and riboflavin, but hogs are most efficient in converting feed into fat, thiamine, and niacin.   The measure of average output of all nutrients indicates that the total quantity of food obtained from feed is greatest when used to produce milk, followed in order by hogs, poultry, and beef cattle.   The value of nonfood byproducts, such as hides from cattle and wool from sheep, should be taken into account but adjustments to allow for these would not greatly affect these conclusions.

TABLE 5.—*Average outputs of food nutrients per 1,000 units of feed used to produce specified livestock products in terms of the number of days that a moderately active man can be supplied with a daily allowance* [1]

Farm product and food use	Food energy	Pro-tein	Fat	Cal-cium	5 vita-mins [2]	10 nu-trients [3]
	Days	*Days*	*Days*	*Days*	*Days*	*Days*
Milk, whole_____	83	181	188	535	105	153
Eggs_____	37	128	108	47	67	81
Chickens_____	27	121	70	8	49	54
Turkeys_____	35	116	108	6	47	60
Hogs_____	116	82	486	5	64	109
Cattle, all_____	21	60	69	3	37	39

[1] See footnote 1 of table 4 for explanation and tables 24 and 25 for more detailed data about these and other products.
[2] See footnote 2 of table 4.
[3] See footnote 3 of table 4.

These comparisons indicate that the production of food nutrients could be increased by shifting feed from poultry, beef cattle, and sheep to milk cows and hogs.   Most of the feed consumed by beef cattle and sheep is not suitable for consumption by hogs, however, and could not readily be shifted to milk cows.   Grains and grain concentrates make up only 6 percent of all the feed now going to sheep and only 20 percent of all the feed going to beef cattle.   Moreover, a large proportion of the roughage feed is from pasture—80 percent for sheep and 70 percent for beef cattle.   Only in the case of livestock-fattening operations can feed now fed to meat animals readily be shifted to hog or dairy production.

The outputs shown in table 5 (and later in table 24) are based upon national average relationships of food from feed.   But the quantity of food obtained from feed depends upon the intensity of feeding and the weight to which meat animals are fed.   Experimental results indicate that more protein food can be produced from feed used to produce milk even when production per cow is raised to a very high level by heavy feeding than from feed used to produce beef cattle or hogs (1), (13), (22).   Fattening of beef cattle provides a little less protein food per unit of feed than do hogs of the average weights to which they usually are fed.   But hogs are the most efficient sources of fat regardless of the intensity of feeding or the weight to which meat animals are fed.   (See table 25 for detailed comparisons.)

Closely related to the efficiency of livestock in converting feed into food is the problem of how land can be used to maximize feed production.   The roughage-consuming livestock (cattle and sheep) compare more favorably in relation to the grain-consuming livestock (hogs and poultry) in food output from feed than in food output from land. This is because feed production per acre, with the present pattern of land use, averages more for the grain crops than for the roughage crops.   But the land used to grow corn and other grains generally is more productive and is fertilized more heavily.   More feed probably can be produced in the United States, especially over a period of some years, by changing the crop pattern to include more roughage crops and less grain, although this is a question that requires more study before an adequate statement can be made.   Especially important are the effects on soil conservation of growing more hay and pasture and the possibilities of raising yields of roughage and grain crops through the development of better plant varieties and the use of more fertilizer.

Food Production per Day of Farm Labor

As national estimates of the farm labor required to produce different products are available, the efficiency of farm products in using labor to produce food can be compared.[18]   The number of days that a moderately active man can be supplied with a daily allowance of each of the food nutrients from an 8-hour day of farm labor used to produce selected products is shown in table 6 (and later in tables 26, 27, 28, and 29).   The data for livestock products include the labor used to produce feed crops.   Field crops and certain vegetables have the highest outputs of nutrients per day of farm labor.   But milk used in whole form is a more efficient source of protein, calcium, and riboflavin than are many of the food crops.   Hogs provide a relatively high output of fat, thiamine, and niacin, compared with many of the food crops.   Vegetables and fruits do not rank so high in relation to other products as they do in production per acre, but they are the most efficient sources of ascorbic acid and vitamin A.

It must be recognized that the relationships referred to are national averages which do not fit all areas of the country.   The products listed are produced in different areas, and comparisons do not indicate exactly how much food is obtained from the same farm labor when used to produce different products.   Moreover, the supply of labor in an area undoubtedly influences the average labor requirements, and the possibilities of increasing the efficiency with which farm labor is employed differ greatly among farm products and among farm areas.

Food production per day of farm labor is affected by the extent of mechanization, the crop yields, and the rates of production per animal, in the case of milk and eggs.   Less labor is required to produce

---

[18] COOPER, M. R., HOLLEY, W. C., HAWTHORNE, H. W. and WASHBURN, R. S. LABOR REQUIREMENTS FOR CROPS AND LIVESTOCK.   Bur. Agr. Econ.   F. M. 40, 140 pp. 1943.   (Processed.)

the feed fed per unit of livestock production in areas where crop yields are relatively high than in those where yields are relatively low.

TABLE 6.—*Average outputs of food nutrients per 8-hour day of farm labor used to produce specified products in terms of the number of days that a moderately active man can be supplied with a daily allowance* [1]

Farm product and food use	Food energy	Pro-teins	Fat	Cal-cium	5 vita-mins [2]	10 nu-trients [3]
	Days	*Days*	*Days*	*Days*	*Days*	*Days*
Livestock products:						
Milk, whole	22	48	50	142	32	43
Eggs	9	33	28	12	17	21
Chickens	9	41	24	3	17	18
Hogs	52	36	217	2	64	67
Cattle, all	18	51	58	3	31	33
Field crops:						
Wheat, white flour	470	613	47	94	89	205
Corn, cornmeal	231	245	93	42	235	221
Potatoes	95	96	51	46	264	181
Sugar beets, sugar	208	0	0	0	0	22
Beans, dry edible	140	377	23	221	163	261
Peanuts, peanut butter	47	85	146	21	59	63
Vegetables, fresh:						
Beets	28	43	2	63	80	69
Cabbage	59	123	17	358	1, 008	587
Carrots	29	34	8	97	1, 025	542
Lettuce	24	70	10	111	240	158
Onions	59	73	10	146	126	107
Peas, green	15	42	2	12	83	56
Sweet corn	57	84	26	19	159	105
Tomatoes	11	20	5	19	175	100
Fruit, fresh:						
Apples	21	4	5	7	26	19
Oranges	31	23	5	76	287	163
Plums	22	12	3	25	65	44
Strawberries	2	2	1	5	26	15

[1] See footnote 1 of table 4 for explanation and tables 26, 27, 28, and 29, for more detailed data about these and other products.
[2] See footnote 2 of table 4.
[3] See footnote 3 of table 4.

The seasonal distribution of labor required to produce farm products is important. An even distribution throughout the year usually is most desirable. Livestock products that require a relatively large part of all labor directly on livestock and relatively little on feed crops have the most even distribution, whereas labor for food crops is seasonal. Direct labor on livestock is 80 percent of all farm labor used to produce milk; the percentages for other products are 65 percent for poultry and 40 percent for hogs and fattening beef cattle. Farmers generally accept a lower rate of return per hour of labor used to produce products that have a relatively even seasonal distribution of labor because they can get some return during seasons when other alternatives are lacking. For example, the farm value of milk produced per hour of labor averaged about $1 in the 1943–45 period but the farm value of hogs and beef cattle produced per hour averaged about 50 percent higher.

Food Production per Unit of All Farm Resources

Land, labor, and other resources are employed in combination with each other, and it is desirable to measure output of food per unit of all farm resources. If prices and production of products become relatively well adjusted to each other during a period of several years, the average price of each product will tend to equal the marginal cost of the total supply. In other words, price equals (at least approximately) the cost of producing the marginal product or the last unit of the total supply. The price of a product, of course, determines the value of the resources used for its production. Therefore, differences among farm products in the food produced per unit of all farm resources in a period can be estimated approximately by comparing the food contents of a fixed value of each product, for example $10 worth, at prevailing prices. Of course, the relationships indicated would apply only for the volume of production of each product in the period considered.

The number of days that a moderately active man can be supplied with a daily allowance of each of the food nutrients per unit of all farm resources used to produce specified products is shown in table 7 (also in tables 30, 31, 32, and 33).[19]

Certain food crops are the most efficient sources of food energy although they do not rank so high relative to livestock products as in the comparisons involving land and labor. This means that costs of other resources than land and labor are responsible for a larger part of the total farm cost of food crops than of livestock products. Some noteworthy changes within food crops from the previous comparisons also may be mentioned. For example, cereals rank much higher in relation to potatoes, peanuts, and sugar beets as efficient sources of food nutrients from all farm resources than they do from land or labor.

With the exception of a few food crops, milk is the least expensive source of calcium and riboflavin and is a relatively low-cost source of protein. Hogs are the lowest cost source of fat, thiamine, and niacin among livestock products, but several food crops provide more of these nutrients per unit of all farm resources. Certain vegetables and citrus fruit provide ascorbic acid and vitamin A most efficiently. Vegetables and fruits to be canned usually are grown in areas where production costs are relatively low, compared with fresh vegetables, and therefore are lower cost sources of nutrients than are the fresh products. For the same reason, manufactured milk products such as evaporated milk and dried skim milk are a lower cost source of nutrients than is fresh milk.

---

[19] A unit of farm resources is defined as the quantity required to produce $10 worth of the farm product in the 1943–45 period. The measure of farm value used to learn the pounds of farm products produced per $10 paid to farmers is the adjusted value obtained by adding Government payments made to farmers and deducting the farm value of byproducts not used directly as food from the gross value or price of the product. The outputs of food shown, therefore, represent those produced per $10 paid for the use of the farm resources actually used to produce them. Payments to farmers per unit of farm product were more stable in past periods, such as 1935–39, but 1943–45 payments are more applicable for the volume of production of each product we have had in recent years. A detailed explanation of how the adjusted farm values for farm products are computed is given in Misc. Pub. 576 (*33*). Current data are shown in THE MARKETING AND TRANSPORTATION SITUATION, BUREAU OF AGRICULTURAL ECONOMICS.

TABLE 7.—*Average outputs of food nutrients per unit of all farm resources used to produce specified products in terms of the number of days that a moderately active man can be supplied with a daily allowance* [1]

Farm product and food use	Food energy	Pro- tein	Fat	Cal- cium	5 vita- mins [2]	10 nu- trients [3]
Livestock products:	*Days*	*Days*	*Days*	*Days*	*Days*	*Days*
Milk, whole	22	49	51	144	32	43
Eggs	8	29	24	11	15	18
Chickens	6	28	17	2	11	13
Hogs	40	28	168	2	50	52
Cattle, all	14	38	43	2	23	25
Field crops:						
Wheat, white flour	205	267	21	41	39	82
Corn, corn meal	248	265	101	46	253	239
Potatoes	40	41	2	20	112	75
Sugar beets, sugar	158	0	0	0	0	17
Beans, dry edible	80	217	14	128	94	150
Peanuts, peanut butter	65	118	201	29	81	87
Vegetables, fresh:						
Beets	31	46	2	69	87	75
Cabbage	15	30	4	89	251	146
Carrots	20	25	5	69	728	386
Lettuce	4	10	2	17	36	24
Onions	20	25	3	49	42	36
Peas, green	9	24	1	7	49	32
Sweet corn	14	20	6	4	38	25
Tomatoes	4	7	2	7	65	37
Fruit, fresh:						
Apples	15	3	4	5	18	13
Oranges	17	13	3	41	156	89
Plums	9	5	1	11	28	19
Strawberries	2	2	1	6	32	18

[1] See footnote 1 of table 4 for explanation and tables 30, 31, 32, and 33 for more detailed data about these and other products.
[2] See footnote 2 of table 4.
[3] See footnote 3 of table 4.

FOOD PRODUCTION PER UNIT OF ALL RESOURCES

As costs of making food available at retail after products leave farms are responsible for nearly half of the total cost of food at retail, it is desirable to measure differences among foods in the efficiency with which they use all resources, nonfarm as well as farm, to produce food nutrients and make them available to consumers (*33*). Following the same procedure as was used for farm resources, the value of a food product at retail may be assumed to represent the value of all the resources used in its production. Differences among foods in the efficiency with which they use all resources to make food available at retail, then, can be measured by the output of nutrients obtained from a fixed value of each product.

The numbers of days that a moderately active man can be supplied with a daily allowance of each of the food nutrients per unit of all farm and nonfarm resources used to produce specified products are shown in table 8 (and in tables 34, 35, 36, and 37).[20]

TABLE 8.—*Average outputs of food nutrients per unit of all farm and nonfarm resources used to produce specified products in terms of the number of days that a moderately active man can be supplied with a daily allowance*[1]

Farm product and food use	Food energy	Pro-tein	Fat	Cal-cium	5 vita-mins [2]	10 nu-trients [3]
Livestock products:	*Days*	*Days*	*Days*	*Days*	*Days*	*Days*
Milk, whole	14	31	32	92	21	28
Eggs	6	22	18	8	11	14
Chickens	4	19	11	1	8	8
Hogs	27	19	115	1	34	35
Cattle, all	9	26	30	1	15	16
Field crops:						
Wheat, white flour	93	121	9	19	17	37
Corn, corn meal	104	111	42	19	107	100
Potatoes	24	24	1	11	65	44
Sugar beets, sugar	74	0	0	0	0	8
Beans, dry edible	51	139	9	82	60	96
Peanuts, peanut butter	31	56	96	14	39	42
Vegetables, fresh:						
Beets	8	12	1	19	23	20
Cabbage	6	12	2	34	96	56
Carrots	8	9	2	26	278	147
Lettuce	2	5	1	8	17	11
Onions	9	11	1	22	19	16
Peas, green	4	10	(4)	3	19	13
Sweet corn	6	8	2	2	15	10
Tomatoes	2	3	1	3	26	15
Fruit, fresh:						
Apples	8	2	2	3	9	7
Oranges	8	6	1	19	71	40
Plums	4	2	(4)	4	11	8
Strawberries	1	1	(4)	2	13	7

[1] See footnote 1 of table 4 for explanation and tables 34, 35, 36, and 37 for more detailed data about these and other products.
[2] See footnote 2 of table 4.
[3] See footnote 3 of table 4.
[4] Less than 0.5.

Products that require considerable processing—cereals, sugar beets, sugarcane, and canned vegetables and fruits—compare less favorably relative to those that require little additional outlay for this purpose than they do in the comparisons involving only farm resources. But the same generalizations about the most efficient sources of each nutrient still apply. It is significant that when the average for the 10 nutrients is used as a measure of total output the differences among

[20] A unit of all farm and nonfarm resources is defined as the quantity required to make $10 worth of the food product available at retail in the 1943–45 period. The measure of retail value used to learn the pounds of food produced per $10 paid by consumers is the adjusted retail value obtained by adding Government payments to farmers and to processors to the gross value or price at retail. The outputs of food shown therefore represent those produced per $10 paid for the use of all the resources used to produce them.

products in the efficiency with which they use resources to produce nutrients are not so great as those indicated by the previous comparisons involving land, farm labor, and all farm resources. For example, milk and hogs provide more food nutrients in relation to their total cost at retail than do many vegetables and fruits and several of the field crops. Of course, it is necessary to rely upon vegetables and fruits for some nutrients such as ascorbic acid and vitamin A but there are decided differences among products within each food group.

These data showing the food nutrients made available for each $10 paid for food at retail indicate how any fixed amount of money can be spent to obtain the most nutrients. Such information is needed by consumers as guides in deciding how adequate diets can be obtained when their purchasing power is definitely limited (31).

RELATIONSHIPS FOR MARGINAL CHANGES IN NATIONAL PRODUCTION

Most of the analysis of the relative efficiency of products as sources of food nutrients thus far has been concerned with national average relationships. But it must be recognized that these relationships may not apply for marginal changes in the national production of individual products. This is demonstrated by the fact that changes in price relationships for products are necessary if changes in the national pattern of farm production and resource use are to be brought about. For example, the price of milk would have to become more favorable relative to prices of other products, such as poultry and meat animals which compete for the same resources, in order to bring about a shift in resources from other products to milk production. If an increase in the price of milk in relation to other products is necessary to bring about an increase in milk production, milk obviously becomes a more expensive source of food nutrients. Food output per unit of resources used in milk production then is reduced relative to other products. Therefore information about the changes in prices required to bring about changes in production or, in other words, data on supply responses, provide a basis for learning what relationships of food output from resources apply for marginal changes in the national output of individual products.

The changes in prices received by farmers that took place together with changes in production of farm products from the average of 1935–39 to 1943 are shown in table 9. Price changes for various livestock products were about the same, but production responded differently. Production of those products that could be expanded most rapidly increased the most. Relatively large increases in production of soybeans, peanuts, and flax were associated with large increases in prices of these products.

In order to decide at least approximately what relationships would apply for future changes in food production, the results of two Nation-wide studies showing the changes in production and consumption that would be associated with changes in prices of individual farm products are summarized in table 9. One study gives estimates of prices and production of farm products that would be required under specified full-employment conditions (39). The estimates are for 1950, which allows time for adjustments to the assumed price conditions to take place. The other gives estimates of the production that would be possible, with assumed farm prices, if farmers put into effect more efficient production methods that would be profitable, and at the same time follow farming methods that would conserve soil resources (*38*).

Each of these studies provides only one estimate of the change in production in response to price for each farm product. It would be necessary to know how production of each product can be expected to respond to other price changes if very specific conclusions are to be drawn about changes in average relationships of food from resources as the national production of individual products changes. But some conclusions can be drawn from these data.

The production changes from 1943 to postwar include increases in milk, beef cattle, lambs, vegetables, and fruits and decreases in chickens, hogs, flaxseed, soybeans, and dry beans (table 9). Price reductions generally are greater for crop products than for livestock, which means that the crop foods would become cheaper relative to livestock products as sources of food nutrients than they were in 1943. As the price of milk declines less than do prices of other livestock products, milk would become more expensive relative to other livestock products as a source of nutrients. Relatively large increases in the production of vegetables and fruit would occur despite a considerable reduction in prices; this indicates that they can be made available in larger quantities without becoming more expensive to consumers.

RESOURCES USED TO PRODUCE THE NATIONAL DIET

To present a general picture of how resources are used to produce food products, estimates of the percentage distribution of resources among the major food groups included in the 1943–45 average civilian diet are shown in table 10. National average relationships of food outputs from resource inputs were used in making these estimates. (See tables 20 to 37.) These average relationships were used for all the food consumed if a part of the supply is produced in the United States, although imports of some products, especially sugar, are important. In addition to the food consumed by civilians, food for noncivilian uses and nonfood products such as cotton and tobacco came from our agricultural resources. But because the foods used for noncivilian purposes, especially military, did not differ greatly from those consumed by civilians, these percentage estimates also indicate fairly accurately how all resources used in food production were allocated among food groups.

The equivalent of nearly 2.7 acres of cropland was used to produce the 1943–45 average civilian diet. Pasture was converted to a cropland equivalent acreage by computing the acreage of tame hay required to produce a quantity of feed equivalent to that obtained from pasture. About 35 percent of the feed consumed by livestock was from pasture, and it accounts for about one-third or 0.9 acres of 2.7 acres of cropland equivalent. About 88 percent or 2.3 acres of the 2.7 acres was used to grow feed for livestock and only 12 percent to grow food crops for direct consumption. This division of cropland equivalent between livestock and food crops takes into account the fact that land used to produce crops for direct human consumption such as wheat, corn, and vegetable oils also provide byproduct feeds that are fed to livestock. A part of the acreage used to grow these crops is charged to livestock.

TABLE 9.—*Percentage changes in farm prices and in production of farm products, average 1935–39 to annual 1943, and 1943 to postwar estimates, that would be associated with specified full-employment conditions and with improved farm production techniques, United States* [1]

Product	1935–39 to 1943		1935–39 to postwar			1943 to postwar		
	Prices	Production	Prices	Production with Full employment	Production with Improved techniques	Prices	Production with Full employment	Production with Improved techniques
	Percent	*Percent*	*Percent*	*Percent*	*Percent*	*Percent*	*Percent*	*Percent*
Livestock products:								
Milk	70	14	60	24	43	−7	9	26
Eggs	76	49	38	30	51	−22	−13	1
Chickens	60	64	33	55	50	−17	−6	−9
Turkeys	76	33	53	106	153	−13	55	90
Hogs	65	82	36	66	63	−18	−10	−11
Beef cattle	81	21	57	25	34	−13	3	10
Lambs	65	27	47	25	50	−11	−9	−9
Wool	75	5	67	9	1	−5	4	−4
Crops:								
Corn	72	31	38	24	40	−20	−5	7
Wheat	68	11	36	3	20	−19	−7	9
Rice	144	30	16	0	28	−52	−23	−2
Soybeans	109	245	95	221	180	−7	−7	−19
Flaxseed	72	373	36	127	155	−20	−52	−46
Peanuts	133	78	67	61	112	−29	−17	9
Potatoes	87	30	43	−3	46	−24	−25	13
Dry beans	76	43	38	16	39	−22	−22	−6
Truck crops	---	---	---	32	51	---	22	39
Oranges	136	49	79	64	---	−24	---	---
All citrus fruit	---	---	---	---	80	---	9	21
Apples	202	---	103	---	---	−33	---	---

All other fruit	------	-12	------	12	12	------	27	27
Sugar	------	-23	------	11	28	------	44	67
Cotton lint	100	-13	30	3	14	-35	18	31
Tobacco	101	-4	79	46	41	-15	52	47
All farm products	80	28	54	35	43	-15	5	12

[1] Estimates for postwar with specified full-employment conditions are from tables 1 and 2 of WHAT PEACE CAN MEAN TO AMERICAN FARMERS (39) and for postwar with full improved farm-production techniques are from tables 2, 16, and 23 of PEACETIME ADJUSTMENTS IN FARMING (38). The postwar prices are the same for identical products except in the latter study, in which prices for milk and potatoes 70 percent higher than the 1935–39 average were used. The postwar data are not forecasts, but are estimates of changes that would be expected under specified conditions.

TABLE 10.—*Estimated percentage distribution of resources used to produce the average 1943–45 civilian diet and total supply of nutrients, by product groups, United States*

Food group	Percentage distribution of resources [1]					Percentage of all nutrients [3]
	Feed	Cropland [2]	Farm labor	All farm resources	All farm and nonfarm resources	
	Percent	*Percent*	*Percent*	*Percent*	*Percent*	*Percent*
Dairy products, excluding butter	20. 9	19. 1	24. 8	24. 7	21. 7	20. 9
Eggs	8. 0	6. 5	9. 7	9. 4	6. 5	3. 7
Meat and poultry	60. 8	53. 3	31. 4	30. 7	26. 3	20. 9
Fats and oils [4]	10. 3	9. 8	15. 0	6. 8	6. 9	6. 1
Dry beans, peas, and nuts	--------	. 7	1. 0	1. 2	1. 3	3. 4
Potatoes and sweet-potatoes	--------	. 8	1. 9	3. 6	3. 5	6. 7
Grain products	--------	7. 1	3. 2	3. 6	5. 9	16. 7
Sugar	--------	. 3	3. 3	2. 3	2. 8	2. 2
Vegetables	--------	1. 5	3. 9	9. 0	14. 4	[5] 19. 4
Fruit	--------	. 9	5. 8	8. 7	10. 7	--------
Total	100. 0	100. 0	100. 0	100. 0	100. 0	100. 0

[1] Resource requirements were computed with the use of national average relationships of food products from resources shown in tables 20 to 37. Resources required to produce the average diet were as follows: 3,160 feed units, 2.67 acres of cropland (including the cropland equivalent of feed from pasture, ten 8-hour days of farm labor, $120 worth of all farm resources, and $225 worth of all farm and nonfarm resources. See footnote 19, p. 31 and footnote 20, p. 33 for definitions of all farm and all farm and nonfarm resources. Resource requirements for products that are imported, such as sugar, are included if a part of the supply is produced in the United States, but requirements for products not produced here, such as coffee and cocoa, are excluded.

[2] Pasture was converted to a cropland-equivalent basis by computing the acreage of tame hay required to provide the feed equivalent supplied by pasture.

[3] Average of 10 nutrients shown in table 11. Individual nutrients are weighted in the proportions they were consumed.

[4] All fats and oils including butter and lard but excluding fat cuts.

[5] Total for vegetables and fruit.

Approximately ten 8-hour days of farm labor were required to produce the average diet consumed in recent years. Farm labor was divided about the same way as land, about 75 percent being devoted to feed-crop and livestock production and 25 percent to food crops. Labor used to produce livestock products is divided about equally between feed crops and direct labor on livestock. These estimates do not include the farm labor that may have been used on pasture. They do not include the labor that was required for maintenance and repair of buildings, fences, and machinery and to produce feed crops for horses and mules. Besides food for domestic consumption, farm labor was used to produce food products for export and nonfood products.

Payments to farmers for the farm commodities that supplied the average civilian diet in 1943–45 averaged about $120 per person; the annual value of these products as bought at retail averaged about $225. If the value of a product during the 1943–45 period is used as a measure of the resources used in its production, 70 percent of all farm resources were devoted to livestock products and 30 percent to food crops. In the case of all farm and nonfarm resources used to make the diet available at retail, the division was about 60 percent for livestock products and 40 percent for foods from crops. This means that a larger proportion of the total value of crop foods at retail is due to marketing costs than is true for livestock products. Payments to farmers for the products from which the average national diet was derived amounted to 53 percent of the total retail value of the diet. This indicates that costs of marketing food were almost as great as the costs of production on the farms.

Estimates of the percentage distribution of resources among food groups are especially significant when compared with percentage estimates of the total consumption of individual nutrients obtained from each group as shown in table 11. For example, grain products provided more than one-fourth of the food energy, protein, iron, thiamine, and niacin contained in the national diet but used only 7 percent of the cropland and 3 percent of the farm labor. Dry beans and peas and potatoes and sweetpotatoes also are definitely efficient sources of food energy and several other nutrients in relation to the resources used for their production. Vegetables and fruit are not so efficient as sources of food energy but provide a relatively large part of the vitamin A and ascorbic acid in relation to the resources they use. Dairy products, excluding butter, supplied one-fourth of the protein, three-fourths of the calcium, and nearly one-half of the riboflavin, and they used one-fifth of the cropland and one-fourth of the farm labor. Meat, poultry, and eggs are less efficient sources of food nutrients as they used about one-half of the cropland and one-third of the farm labor to provide 14 percent of the food energy and 35 percent of the protein, but they are notable sources of iron, thiamine, and niacin. Fats and oils and sugar are important from a dietary standpoint mainly as sources of food energy.

The percentage distribution of resources among product groups also can be compared with the percentages of all nutrients obtained from each group shown in the last column of table 10. These percentages are simple averages of the percentages for all 10 nutrients shown in table 11. This has the effect of weighting the nutrients in the proportions in which they were consumed. Grain products, potatoes and sweetpotatoes, and dry beans and peas, provide the most nutrients in relation to the resources used in their production. Dairy products, excluding butter, rank next. Meat, poultry, and eggs are relatively expensive sources of food nutrients. Vegetables and fruits are efficient sources of several nutrients, especially vitamin A and ascorbic acid, but they are relatively expensive sources of all nutrients considered together.

TABLE 11.—*Percentage of total nutrients contributed by major food groups to the 1944–45 average civilian diet, United States* [1]

Food group	Calories	Protein	Fat	Calcium	Iron
	Percent	Percent	Percent	Percent	Percent
Dairy products, excluding butter_____	13. 7	24. 0	18. 6	74. 3	3. 3
Eggs_____	2. 3	7. 0	4. 3	2. 4	7. 6
Meat, poultry, game, fish_____	11. 5	28. 0	22. 1	1. 9	23. 4
Fats and oils, including fat cuts and butter_____	18. 3	2. 0	48. 6	. 4	1. 1
Dry beans, peas, nuts, and soya flour__	2. 8	5. 0	2. 9	2. 2	7. 1
Potatoes and sweetpotatoes_____	3. 9	3. 0	(2)	1. 9	5. 4
Citrus fruit and tomatoes_____	1. 4	1. 0	(2)	2. 2	3. 3
Leafy, green, yellow vegetables_____	1. 4	2. 0	(2)	4. 9	6. 5
Other vegetables and fruit_____	4. 1	2. 0	. 7	4. 0	7. 1
Grain products_____	26. 5	26. 0	2. 1	4. 5	28. 2
Sugar and sirups_____	13. 6	(2)	0	1. 3	6. 5
Cocoa_____	. 5	(2)	. 7	0	. 5
Total_____	100. 0	100. 0	100. 0	100. 0	100. 0

Food group	Vitamin A	Thiamine	Riboflavin	Niacin	Ascorbic acid
	Percent	Percent	Percent	Percent	Percent
Dairy products, excluding butter_____	11. 7	9. 9	44. 8	3. 3	5. 8
Eggs_____	5. 9	2. 7	6. 4	(2)	0
Meat, poultry, game, fish_____	7. 6	25. 6	16. 0	40. 4	1. 4
Fats and oils, including fat cuts and butter_____	5. 9	3. 6	. 8	1. 9	0
Dry beans, peas, nuts, and soya flour__	. 1	4. 5	2. 0	7. 0	(2)
Potatoes and sweetpotatoes_____	16. 4	6. 7	2. 4	7. 5	18. 9
Citrus fruit and tomatoes_____	7. 5	3. 1	1. 6	2. 8	29. 7
Leafy, green, yellow vegetables_____	35. 4	5. 8	4. 8	3. 3	28. 3
Other vegetables and fruit_____	9. 1	4. 5	4. 0	4. 7	15. 9
Grain products_____	. 4	33. 6	16. 0	28. 1	0
Sugar and sirups_____	0	(2)	. 4	. 5	(2)
Cocoa_____	0	(2)	. 8	. 5	0
Total_____	100. 0	100. 0	100. 0	100. 0	100. 0

[1] From CLARK, FRIEND, and BURK (*4, p. 22*).
[2] Less than 0.05 percent.

RESOURCE REQUIREMENTS FOR DIFFERENT DIETS

Because of the wide variations in output of food nutrients from resources used to produce different products, the total population that can be supported with available resources depends upon the make-up of the diet. This is illustrated by data in table 12, showing the acres of land required to produce the average 1943–45 civilian diet and three different cost diets and the number of people that could be supported with each diet, assuming average yields. The three different-cost diets provide at least the National Research Council's recommended allowances of each nutrient, but the most expensive would satisfy preferences most fully. It includes more livestock products, citrus fruit, and certain vegetables, and less cereals and potatoes, than do the lower-cost diets.   The relative importance of livestock products and crop foods is indicated by the percentage of all food energy obtained from livestock products.

TABLE 12.—*Acres of cropland required to produce different-cost adequate diets, the number of people that can be supported with each diet, and the percentage of food energy from livestock products in each diet, United States* [1]

Diet plan	Cropland required per person [2]	Number of people that can be supported [3]	Food energy in diet from livestock
	Acres	*Millions*	*Percent*
Low-cost_____	2. 12	203	30
Moderate-cost_____	2. 57	167	36
Liberal-cost_____	3. 15	137	44
1943–45 civilian diet_____	2. 67	161	38

[1] The different-cost adequate diets are those described by the UNITED STATES BUREAU OF HUMAN NUTRITION AND HOME ECONOMICS PLANNING DIETS IN NEW YARDSTICK OF FOOD NUTRITION; LOW COST, MODERATE COST, AND LIBERAL.   14 pp., 1941.   (Processed.)   These diets provide a fairly high level of nutrition.   The liberal diet includes more of the products relatively expensive as sources of food nutrients than does the low-cost.

[2] All cropland when pasture is converted to a cropland-equivalent basis by computing the acreage of tame hay that would be required to provide a quantity of feed equivalent to that supplied by pasture.   Average 1941–45 crop yields were used.

[3] These numbers are based on a total cropland equivalent of 430 million acres. This includes 355 million acres of harvested crops, minus 30 million acres of nonfood and nonfeed crops and 35 million acres of feed crops for horses, plus 140 million acres as an allowance for the cropland-equivalent of feed from pasture.   Total civilian population in United States averaged 129.5 millions in 1943–45, but only 80 percent of the total food supply was used by civilians.

If average yields apply for changes in production of individual products, about 200 million people could be supported with the low-cost diet, about 170 million with the moderate, and about 140 million with the liberal diet, from present land resources.   These figures may be compared with the estimate of about 160 million which could be supported with the average 1943–45 civilian diet.   The actual population of the United States was 140 million in 1945, but a part of the total population was in the military services and nearly 20 percent of all food supplies was exported or used for noncivilian purposes. Considerable growth in the population of the United States is expected in the years ahead.   But it should be apparent that many more people could be supported with adequate diets, without employing additional resources (even though greater efficiencies in the use of resources do not take place), by changing the national pattern of resource use to include more crop foods and less livestock products. Of course, shifts in consumption of foods would be required.

Improvement in the quality of the national diet can provide market outlets for all the food that can be produced.   This is apparent from table 13, which shows the cropland required to produce the average diet consumed by different income groups in 1942 (*34*). About 2.5 acres was required per person to produce the average diet of all income groups as compared with an average of 2.7 acres in 1943–45, but food consumption per capita based on disappearance data was about 6 percent less in 1942 than in 1943–45. More than 200 million people could be supported with the average diet consumed by consumption units (families and single persons) whose net money income was less than $500 per year. On the other hand, only about 140 million persons could be supported with the average diet consumed by those in consumption units with incomes of $3,000 or more per year.

People who have relatively high incomes consume much larger quantities of livestock products and only slightly less of the crop foods than do those in the low-income groups. As a result, the quantity of resources used to produce the diets consumed by people in the various income groups differ greatly. Land requirements for livestock products are relatively high in the case of the diets of those in the high-income groups, whereas requirements for crop foods do not differ much. About 50 percent more land, 70 percent more farm labor, and 65 percent more of all farm resources were required to produce the average diet consumed by people in consumption units (families and single persons) which had an annual money income larger than $3,000 than were required for the diets of those in consumption units with an annual money income of less than $500.

TABLE 13.—*Acres of cropland required to produce the average diet consumed by different income groups and the number of people that could be supported from present land resources with present production rates, United States* [1]

Net money income class (dollars) [2]	Cropland requirements for [3]—			Number of people that could be supported with each diet [4]
	All food products	Livestock products	Food crops	
	Acres	*Acres*	*Acres*	*Millions*
Under 500	1. 90	1. 52	0. 38	226
500–999	2. 13	1. 77	. 36	202
1,000–1,499	2. 31	1. 98	. 33	186
1,500–1,999	2. 54	2. 23	. 31	169
2,000–2,999	2. 83	2. 53	. 30	152
3,000 and over	3. 03	2. 75	. 28	142
All classes	2. 51	2. 19	. 32	171

[1] Average diets consumed by people in each net money income class in 1942 as reported by the Bureau of Human Nutrition and Home Economics (*34*).

[2] Net money income per year of the consumption unit, family or single person.

[3] All cropland when pasture is converted to a cropland-equivalent basis by computing the acreage of tame hay required to provide a quantity of feed equivalent to that supplied by pasture. Average 1941–45 crop yields were used.

[4] These numbers are based on a total cropland equivalent of 430 million acres. This includes 355 million acres of harvested crops, minus 30 million acres of nonfood and nonfeed crops and 35 million acres of feed crops for horses plus 140 million acres as an allowance for the cropland equivalent of feed from pasture.

These comparisons indicate that it is readily possible from a physical standpoint to consume, by improving the quality of diets, all the commodities that can be produced with the resources now used in food production at present production rates.   Moreover, the comparisons indicate that food production would have to be increased if it is to provide all of our people with a diet like that of people in the high-income groups.   For example, approximately 30 percent more food would have been consumed if all people had diets like those of people in consumption units that received money incomes over $3,000 in 1942.   This would be equivalent to a per capita consumption of food about 35 percent higher than the 1935-39 average.   To make possible this rate of consumption for the 1946 population of 141 million, the total volume of food production would have to be about 10 percent higher than the recent 1942-45 wartime average.

FOOD PRODUCTION AND CONSUMPTION AHEAD

POSSIBLE PRODUCTION CHANGES

It is apparent from the detailed information that has been presented concerning the relative efficiency of products as sources of nutrients that there are many ways in which food production and consumption could be changed to supply the additional nutrients that may be needed to provide better diets.   But not all of the possible consumption changes would satisfy tastes and preferences of consumers equally well.   With respect to this, Maynard recently said that—

milk, eggs, and fruit, and to a lesser extent, the nutritious vegetables are the preferred foods.   Nutrition is best served when foods which are most nutritious and most highly prized are available in abundance.   Food habits are of tremendous importance.   Changes can be brought about only very slowly when shifts to the less preferred foods of lower nutritional quality are involved (15, p. 322).

The extent to which desires of consumers for food can be met in the future depends upon per capita consumption that will be possible, and this in turn depends upon the total volume of food production. Future changes in production undoubtedly will be influenced by changes in the demand for farm products.   The following estimates by T. W. Schultz with respect to prospective changes in the first decade after the war are illustrative.

With farm prices averaging at least parity (as parity is now defined by law), an increase in agricultural production of as much as 20 percent over the wartime level (1942–45 average) may be expected * * *.   Even with farm prices as low as 75 percent of parity, some increase in agricultural production may be expected, possibly as little as 5 percent but more likely nearer 10 percent (24, p. 81).

Parity prices as defined by existing legislation may be described briefly as prices received for farm products relative to prices paid by farmers the same as during a base period.   For most farm products this period is 1910–14.

Agricultural production undoubtedly will be larger if farm prices continue to average above parity as they did during the recent war years than if they decline.   But it is doubtful that production will be reduced even if prices decline substantially.   The recent expansion in farm output was achieved mainly by improved production methods which result in more efficient use of resources and in reduced costs per unit of product.   Most of these methods do not involve much or any additional cash outlay and will presumably be profitable to farmers even though farm prices decline.

As the volume of food production in the future cannot be regarded as fixed, it is desirable to consider consumption possibilities in connection with different levels of production. The possibilities of expanding production within the next few years were examined in detail in a recent study (38). It was estimated that the wartime volume of farm output could be increased about 10 percent if improved production methods were adopted to the extent they would be profitable if farm prices average parity and if necessary soil-conserving practices were put into effect. This estimate was not a forecast but an appraisal of what would be possible under specified conditions. A 10-percent increase in food output from the 1943–45 average may be considered the maximum possible by 1955.

At the opposite extreme is the possibility that food production will not increase but will remain the same as in the 1943–45 period.

Midway between these two is the possibility that food production will increase 5 percent. This is the same as the increase in agricultural production which was estimated in the study of agriculture under specified full employment conditions as necessary to supply demand at farm prices averaging parity (39).

These three levels of food production would make possible different levels of per capita consumption for the population expected in 1955. If exports and imports of food products are the same percentage of total food production in 1955 as in the 1935–39 period, per capita consumption could be increased 5 percent, 10 percent, or 15 percent from the 1942–45 wartime average (table 14).

TABLE 14.—*Total population, total food production, food production per capita, and food consumption per capita, United States, averages 1941–45, 1942–45, and 1943–45, annual 1946, and estimates for 1955 (index numbers, 1935–39=100)*

Item	Averages			1946	1955 possibilities [1]		
	1941–45	1942–45	1943–45		1	2	3
Total population [2]	106	106	107	109	118	118	118
Total food production [3]	130	133	136	139	136	143	150
Food production per capita	123	126	127	127	115	121	127
Food consumption per capita [4]	110	110	111	118	115	121	127

[1] The possibilities considered here are no change, a 5-percent increase, and a 10-percent increase in total food production from the 1943–45 volume. If exports and imports are the same percentage of total food production in 1955 as in 1935–39, the food supply available for consumption would be great enough, with the indicated changes in production, to make possible increases of 5, 10, and 15 percent, respectively, in food consumption per capita from the 1941–45 or 1942–45 averages. The data shown are not forecasts but are indications of the possibilities with respect to food production and consumption under specified conditions described in the text.

[2] A United States population estimate of 153 million was used for 1955. This would allow an increase of 8 million from the 1948 population of 145 million, or approximately 1 million per year.

[3] Volume of food production for sale and farm home consumption.

[4] Food consumption per capita by civilians, 1941–46, and by total population, 1955.

More food will be available for domestic use if foreign trade returns to prewar levels.   Imports of food (including products not produced in the United States such as coffee, tea, and bananas) exceeded exports in the 1935–39 period, and net imports were equivalent to 4.5 percent of domestic food production.   We shifted to a net export basis during the war, and in the 1942–45 period net exports were equivalent to about 3 percent of food production.   Exports of food products continued to exceed total imports in 1946 and 1947.   Exports undoubtedly will remain high during the next few years because of food shortages in other countries, but they probably will decline again as production in foreign areas recovers from the effects of war.

POSSIBLE CONSUMPTION CHANGES

In each of the production situations described above, there would be alternative ways in which national consumption of food products could be changed to provide the additional nutrients that were estimated earlier as necessary to raise all diets that are below a specified level of adequacy to such a level.   To learn which of these would satisfy desires of consumers most fully, differences in consumption among people in different income groups may be examined.   Such information indicates what products and how much of each our people would buy in larger or smaller quantities if their purchasing power were increased.

The changes in food consumption that people prefer to make are suggested by data from the 1942 survey of food consumption summarized in table 15 (*34*).   The foods that would be consumed in larger quantities if incomes were increased are dairy products, eggs, meat, poultry, vegetables, and fruit.   Consumption of sugar and fats and potatoes would not change materially, and consumption of dry beans and peas, and grain products, would be reduced.   It should be recognized that the selection of food products depends upon their prices and that the data in table 15 indicate the changes in consumption which people probably would make if their incomes increased while prices remained the same as in 1942.

These national-average data by food groups conceal some significant differences in consumption among the various income and population groups.   Home-produced foods, which account for about half of all the food consumed by rural people of course are available to them at much lower prices than are similar foods to urban people.   Because the value of home-produced and consumed foods is not counted as income in the classification followed, a larger proportion of rural people are included in the lower income classes than otherwise would be the case.   Therefore, the changes in food consumption that occur as incomes increase are greater than are indicated by these national averages.   The changes in food consumption that people would prefer to make if their incomes were increased are indicated more accurately by consumption data for urban groups, who depend almost entirely on purchased foods.   Urban people with high incomes consume more than twice as much whole milk, butter, meat, citrus fruit, and certain vegetables per capita than do those with relatively low incomes.   But people with low incomes consume much more evaporated milk, salt pork, lard, dry beans and peas, and flour and meal.

TABLE 15.—*Average quantity of specified groups of food consumed at home per household per week and average size of household classified by net money income of household, United States* [1]

Food group and average size of household	Food consumed per household and size of household with income of—					
	Under $500	$500– $999	$1,000– $1,499	$1,500– $1,999	$2,000– $2,999	$3,000 and over
	Pounds	*Pounds*	*Pounds*	*Pounds*	*Pounds*	*Pounds*
Dairy products (excluding butter)	28. 5	26. 9	29. 3	31. 3	30. 7	34. 6
Eggs	2. 5	2. 8	3. 3	3. 6	3. 7	3. 8
Meat, poultry, and fish	4. 1	5. 7	6. 8	7. 6	9. 7	11. 9
Fats and oils (including fat cuts and butter)	3. 8	3. 9	4. 0	4. 0	3. 8	4. 3
Dry beans, peas, and nuts	1. 5	1. 3	1. 5	1. 0	1. 0	. 9
Potatoes and sweetpotatoes	8. 4	8. 9	10. 5	9. 9	9. 8	10. 2
Citrus fruit and tomatoes	4. 1	6. 1	7. 5	8. 8	11. 7	14. 7
Leafy, green, and yellow vegetables	5. 6	6. 1	6. 6	6. 8	8. 0	9. 2
Other vegetables and fruit	7. 0	8. 5	10. 1	10. 1	11. 9	13. 7
Grain products	14. 7	13. 8	12. 4	10. 8	11. 1	11. 2
Sugar and sirups	3. 6	3. 6	3. 6	3. 2	3. 4	3. 4
Total	83. 8	87. 6	95. 6	97. 1	104. 8	117. 9
	Number	*Number*	*Number*	*Number*	*Number*	*Number*
Average size of household in equivalent persons	3. 03	3. 16	3. 37	3. 29	3. 44	3. 80

[1] From Bureau of Human Nutrition and Home Economics (*34*).

The quantities of various foods consumed per person differ considerably among the different income or population groups although total pounds of food is about the same. In general, people with low incomes eat more of the foods relatively low in cost as sources of nutrients. The products they especially desire in larger quantities to satisfy preferences more fully are meat, eggs, milk, fruits, and certain vegetables. These products have a high content of minerals and vitamins in relation to caloric content and could be consumed in larger quantities to improve diets. If this takes place, use of other products such as cereals and potatoes probably would be reduced.

In considering how the national diet can be changed to supply the additional nutrients that may be required to improve diets, it is useful to consider again the percentage contribution of the major food groups to the total consumption of each nutrient (table 11). Dairy products provide three-fourths of the calcium and nearly one-half of the riboflavin contained in the national diet. In examining the possibilities of substituting one product for another to supply the same nutrient, it is soon discovered that few foods can be substituted for dairy products to any great extent as sources of calcium and riboflavin. Although grain products, dry beans and peas, and certain vegetables are lower cost sources of these nutrients, they cannot be relied upon for a very large part of the additional needs because they are bulky, high in caloric content, and not very palatable when eaten in large quantities. Other food nutrients can be obtained from many different products in the quantities required. For example, dry beans and peas, grain products, and potatoes have a relatively high content of thiamine and niacin in relation to caloric content. Meats, poultry, and eggs also are important sources of thiamine and niacin. Vitamin A and ascorbic acid are contained in many foods, especially fruits and vegetables, that are relatively low in energy content.

All of the changes in consumption that would provide the additional needs for minerals and vitamins also would provide adequate supplies of food energy, protein, and fat. The problem is one of learning how the additional minerals and vitamins can be supplied without a greatly increased consumption of calories. This is much easier if products relatively high in cost as sources of energy such as livestock products and certain fruits and vegetables which generally have a high content of minerals and vitamins in relation to caloric content, are consumed in larger quantities. Of course, such changes in consumption also would supply food preferences more fully and so could be achieved more readily.

It now is possible to suggest, at least approximately, how national consumption of foods could be changed to supply the additional nutrients that would be required to improve diets with the kinds of foods, that would involve the least departure from existing food habits and preferences, under the three situations with respect to production and consumption described above (table 14). Changes in per capita consumption from the 1942–45 average which would increase the per capita supply of nutrients by the quantities estimated earlier as desirable to improve diets are shown in table 16.

These are approximate estimates by major food groups, and all products within each group would not have to change by the same percentage. Each set of consumption changes would increase the per capita supply of nutrients by at least the following percentages: calcium 12, vitamin A 10, ascorbic acid 10, niacin 8, iron 7, thiamine 5, riboflavin 5. None of them would involve more than a 5-percent increase in food energy, or a 10-percent increase in total pounds of food per person. The percentage increases in per capita supplies of nutrients listed are those that would be necessary to raise average consumption of nutrients in those income and population groups that were below the content of a low-cost diet in 1942 to this level. (See p. 10.) Of course, consumption of foods could be changed in other ways to supply even greater quantities of nutrients. It should be noted that consumption of many foods was higher in 1946 and 1947 than in the preceding few years, and that the changes described here are from the average of 1942–45.

If the total volume of food production averages 10 percent higher in 1955 than it did in the 1943–45 war years, so that a 15-percent increase in total consumption per capita would be possible, all diets that are inadequate could be raised to an adequate level with the kinds of food that would satisfy preferences relatively well. It would be necessary to increase the consumption of whole-milk products to obtain additional calcium and riboflavin. Citrus fruit and tomatoes would be increased to provide ascorbic acid with products that people would like in larger quantities. Eggs, meats, and vegetables would furnish additional thiamine and niacin and smaller quantities of other nutrients. Consumption of meat, poultry, eggs, and certain dairy

products, which people especially want, would be increased to the
extent possible to satisfy food preferences, although they are not
required in the quantities that are indicated to supply additional
nutrients. Consumption of sugar and fats would be raised to prewar
levels although additional supplies of these products are not required
from a dietary standpoint. Grain products, potatoes, and dry beans
and peas could be reduced because the consumption of food energy
would be more than adequate. In general, the national diet would
become more like that now consumed by people in the high-income
groups.

TABLE 16.—*Per capita food consumption, average 1942–45, and
approximate estimates of changes that would raise all diets to an adequate
level, by major food groups, United States* [1]

Food group	Per capita consumption, average 1942–45 [2]	Percentage changes by food groups if total consumption per capita is increased [3]—		
		5 percent	10 percent	15 percent
	Pounds	*Percent*	*Percent*	*Percent*
Dairy products (excluding butter)[4]	521	15	18	20
Eggs	42	−3	10	20
Meat, poultry, and fish	160	−3	10	20
Fats and oils (including fat cuts and butter)	65	0	3	5
Dry beans, peas, and nuts	21	10	−10	−15
Potatoes and sweetpotatoes	141	10	−10	−15
Citrus fruit and tomatoes	109	10	15	20
Leafy, green, and yellow vegetables	120	20	20	20
Other vegetables and fruit	218	0	10	20
Grain products	205	10	−5	−15
Sugar and sirups	101	0	5	10

[1] These changes in consumption per capita would be possible for the expected
1955 population if total food production changes, as described in table 14. See
text for more detailed explanation of the application of these data.
[2] From THE NATIONAL FOOD SITUATION. Bur. Agr. Econ. 42 pp. October–
December 1947. (Processed.)
[3] The changes in total consumption per capita refer to foods valued at 1935–39
average prices. The changes by food groups refer to pounds of food. Each set
of consumption changes would increase the 1942–45 per capita supply of nutrients
by at least the following percentages: calcium 12, iron 7, vitamin A 10, ascorbic
acid 10, niacin 8, and riboflavin 5. These are estimates of the additional consumption of nutrients that would be required if average consumption of those population
groups that were below the content of a low-cost diet were to be raised to this
level. (See p. 10.) None of the sets of consumption changes would involve more
than a 5-percent increase in food energy or a 10-percent increase in total pounds of
food per person.
[4] Milk equivalent calculated on basis of protein and mineral content.

If food production were increased only 5 percent, so that a 10-
percent increase in per capita consumption would be possible, all
diets could be raised to an adequate level but not with the kinds of
foods that people like as well. It would be necessary to increase the
consumption of whole-milk products, citrus fruit and tomatoes, and

the leafy, green, and yellow vegetables in order to obtain additional supplies of nutrients. It still would be possible to increase consumption of meat, eggs, and the other vegetables and fruits although not as greatly. They could replace some of the grain products, dry beans and peas, and potatoes and sweetpotatoes.

If total food production were not changed and only a 5-percent increase in total consumption per capita is possible, changes in diets that would not satisfy preferences very well would have to be made to increase supplies of nutrients by the required quantities. It still would be necessary to increase the consumption of whole-milk products, citrus fruit and tomatoes, and the leafy, green, and yellow vegetables (table 16). Consumption of grain products would have to be increased but meat, poultry, and eggs would be reduced slightly to make possible certain increases in the other products.

These comparisons show that further expansion in food production is required if we are to provide additional supplies of nutrients in the forms that will involve little change in food habits and will best satisfy food preferences. It would be possible to increase supplies of nutrients by shifting resources to produce more of the products that give a relatively high output of nutrients, but this would involve changes in consumption that people do not prefer to make; it would be difficult to achieve, and it would not be necessary if the volume of food production can be expanded. It is worthy of note that increased production of dairy products, meats, poultry, eggs, fruits, and certain vegetables would make possible a continuation of consumption trends which have resulted in greatly improved diets in recent years.

Somewhat different changes in food consumption from the national averages shown in table 16 would be required by people in the various population groups in order that they receive nutrients in the quantities contained in the low-cost diets. As average consumption of nutrients is lowest among people in the low-income groups, they would have to increase consumption of the foods that have a high content of nutrients such as milk, citrus fruits, and leafy, green, and yellow vegetables more than would people with high incomes. Rural people need to increase consumption of citrus fruits and tomatoes relatively more than other products because their diets are most deficient in ascorbic acid. On the other hand, diets of urban people are most deficient in calcium, and increased consumption of whole-milk products are especially needed to supply these shortages.

ACHIEVING THE CONSUMPTION CHANGES

Expenditures for food would have to average higher than in the 1942–45 war years to make possible the consumption changes that have been described, unless prices of foods were reduced. Starting from data that show how additional consumption of nutrients must be distributed among the different income groups, it would be possible to decide how the national changes in consumption of food products (table 16) need to be distributed if average consumption of nutrients within each group is to be raised to an adequate level. Approximate estimates of the average additional expenditures for food that are necessary by people in each group could then be made. Such estimates are shown in table 17. They are rough approximations because

TABLE 17.—*Approximate estimates of the increases in food expenditures and in income per person that would be required to achieve the consumption changes that would raise average consumption of nutrients within each income group to an adequate level, United States* [1]

Annual net money income of household in 1942 (dollars)	Annual averages per person in 1942–45		Percentage increases in food expenditures if total consumption per capita is increased [4]—			Ratio of change in food expenditure to change in income [5]	Percentage increases in income if total consumption per capita is increased [6]—		
	Food expenditure [2]	Income [3]	5 percent	10 percent	15 percent		5 percent	10 percent	15 percent
	Dollars	Dollars	Percent	Percent	Percent	Percent	Percent	Percent	Percent
0–499	122	251	12	23	34	1.0	12	23	34
500–999	152	447	9	17	26	.9	10	19	29
1,000–1,499	183	650	7	13	20	.8	9	16	25
1,500–1,999	219	857	5	10	15	.7	7	14	21
2,000–2,999	249	1,083	4	8	12	.6	6	12	20
3,000 or over	318	1,994	2	4	7	.5	4	8	14
All groups	222	985	5	10	15	------	6	12	18

[1] See text of this study for more detailed explanation of the application of these data.

[2] Total expenditures for food in 1942–45 (as reported by THE MARKETING AND TRANSPORTATION SITUATION. Bur. Agr. Econ. 21 pp. September 1947) distributed among people in the different income groups in the same way as was the value of food consumption reported in the 1942 study (37, pp. 70–75).

[3] Average national disposable income of 136 billion dollars in 1942–45 distributed among income groups in the same way as was income reported in the 1942 study (37).

[4] Approximate estimates of the increases in food expenditures that would be required, with 1942–45 average prices, to cover the cost of the consumption changes indicated in table 16, if they were distributed among income groups in such a way as to raise average consumption of food nutrients within each income group to an adequate level.

[5] Estimated ratios of percentage changes in food expenditures to percentage changes in income as indicated by data for urban people by HANSEN and CORNFIELD (11, table 7).

[6] Estimates of the average increases in income that would be necessary for food expenditures to increase by the average amounts indicated if the relationships between change in food expenditures and change in income shown apply. Percentage changes for all groups depend upon the number of people in each group.

the detailed data required for making very accurate estimates are
not available, but they can be referred to for illustrative purposes.
It is assumed that additional food is available at no change in prices.
Increases in expenditures differ, depending upon the consumption
plan that is followed or upon the extent to which total consumption
per capita is increased.   But in each instance they are largest for
people who have low incomes because their diets are the most inadequate.

Incomes of consumers also would have to average higher than in
the 1942–45 period before expenditures for food would increase by the
amounts necessary to provide better diets (fig. 8).   According to a

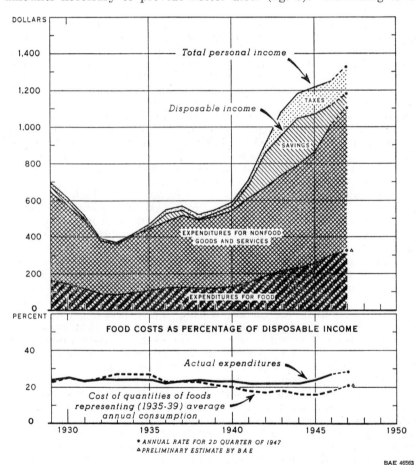

FIGURE 8.—Per capita food costs, expenditures and consumers income, United
States, 1929–47.

recent study, the ratio of a percentage increase in food expenditures
to a percentage increase in net money income varies from slightly
over 1 in the lowest income group to about one-half in the highest (11).
In other words, a small percentage increase in income is accompanied
by about the same percentage increase in expenditures for food when

incomes are very low, but the response declines as incomes increase. On the basis of these relationships, estimates are shown in table 17 of the average percentage increases in income for each income group that would be necessary if expenditures for food were to increase by the amounts required to cover the cost of the additional consumption. The increases that would be required differ considerably depending upon the extent to which per capita consumption is increased or upon the consumption plan that is followed to improve diets. But in each instance, the percentage increases are largest for people who have low incomes because their diets are most deficient; so relatively large additional expenditures for food are necessary to make them adequate.

According to these estimates, incomes would not have to increase greatly, if food prices do not change, to achieve the indicated changes in food expenditures (table 17). To minimize the increases in total income that would be necessary, incomes of people in the low-income groups would have to be increased much more than those of people in the high-income groups. In fact, more equal distribution of the total national income would cause expenditures for food to be increased. Here it should be noted that the distribution of national income has not changed greatly in the past as the national income changed (*11, 18*). However, additions to incomes of people in the different income groups as shown in table 17 would not change substantially the distribution of national income although they would cause demand for food to increase substantially.

It should be recognized that even if incomes were high enough so that expenditures for food would be increased by the amounts necessary, the particular products required to meet nutritional shortages would not be bought, unless food habits and preferences also were modified. Food consumption would be increased and diets would become more like those of people with high incomes. But this does not mean that all would receive adequate diets, for many people with high incomes do not have enough of all nutrients. The extent to which food habits and preferences would have to be modified would depend upon the extent to which per capita consumption of food can be increased or upon the consumption plan that is followed to supply the additional nutrients. For example, they would have to be modified less if total consumption per capita can be increased 15 percent than if it can be increased only 5 percent.

To change food habits and preferences so that adequate diets would be consumed, if the income barrier to additional consumption were removed, more widespread diffusion of knowledge about nutritional requirements for good health and the nutrient content of foods is necessary. The different means for doing this have been discussed fully elsewhere (*19*). The problem is one of creating a greater general recognition of the beneficial effects on health that accrue to the individual and to society as the result of better nutrition. In addition to general education, positive efforts to improve health may be made through public programs. For example, the National School Lunch Program and the industrial in-plant feeding programs, which emphasize the increased consumption of nutritious foods, can be very effective in bringing about better food habits. This is especially true of school lunch programs, which influence food habits in the formative stage. These programs will tend to increase the availability of the foods required for better diets.

Changes in food habits and preferences of course would bring about shifts in demand for food products. Food consumption would be modified regardless of whether prices change. For example, greater recognition of the high nutrient content in relation to cost of whole-milk products and certain vegetables and fruit would cause consumers to buy more of these products and probably less of others. The effects of such developments on the total demand for food cannot be predicted accurately. Some people, especially those with high incomes, might increase their consumption of the highly nutritious foods without reducing their consumption of others. Many might find ways of selecting better diets with the money they now spend for food. In some instances, a better diet might be obtained with smaller expenditures.

It can be concluded that purchasing power of consumers must be increased and food habits and preferences modified before an adequate diet will be consumed by all (*32, p. 168*). Estimates of the increases in purchasing power that would be necessary to achieve desirable consumption changes were indicated by the estimates of increases in food expenditures and in incomes shown in table 17. They assumed no change in prices for foods. But it should be recognized that purchasing power also would be increased if prices were reduced. Therefore, more efficient production and marketing methods, which reduce costs of food products, would help to achieve the consumption changes. They would help to make possible a larger volume of consumption per capita without increasing expenditures for food. Of course, if prices of the foods that are needed in larger quantities to improve diets could be reduced in cost in relation to other foods, consumers would freely select better diets even though their food preferences are not changed.

FUTURE ADJUSTMENTS IN FARM PRODUCTION

Farm production was adjusted to meet changes in food needs that arose during the war from disruption of foreign trade, from increased exports for war purposes, and from increased domestic demand. The volume of farm production was increased about one-third, but demand increased much more, and farm prices doubled (fig. 9).

Price relationships were modified as the pattern of farm production changed and as demand for all products did not increase to the same extent. Demand for food products has changed considerably during the recent period of foreign relief but can be expected to change even more in the future. If foreign trade returns to something like the prewar level, imports would be larger and exports would be smaller than in the last few years. A larger supply of farm products would have to be disposed of in the domestic market. Such developments, together with continued improvement in the methods of farm production, which tend to raise total output, would make adjustments in the present pattern of farm production desirable.

Adjustments in farm production in the future can be considered desirable from at least three standpoints: (1) To improve diets, (2) to supply effective demand as fully as possible, and (3) to maximize net income of farm operators. Achievement of adequate diets for all would require changes in consumption of food products, especially among people with low incomes, which cannot be expected unless incomes are increased and food habits and preferences are modified. If these developments take place, the demand for farm products would be changed from what otherwise could be expected. Diets can be improved and demand met most fully if the total volume of production is increased, but the probable effect on farm income of expanding total output needs to be examined.

FOOD PRODUCTION AND CONSUMPTION COMPARED

To help in deciding what changes in production would be necessary to improve diets, food production in 1946 is compared in table 18 with food requirements from domestic production as they would be in 1955 if per capita consumption were changed as indicated earlier (table 16).

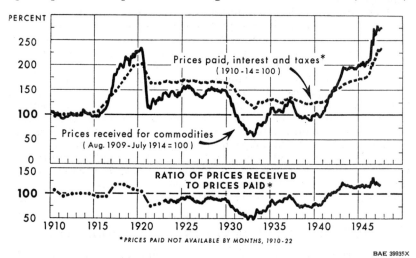

BAE 39935X

FIGURE 9.—Prices received and paid by farmers, index numbers, United States, by months, 1910–47.

The suggested changes depend upon the extent to which the total volume of food production can be increased and more of the foods required to meet desires of consumers can be supplied. The possibilities considered are those mentioned previously—no change, a 5-percent increase, and a 10-percent increase in the 1943–45 average volume of food production. Together with the additional food that would be made available for domestic use if foreign trade returns to prewar levels, these increases would make possible per capita increases in consumption of 5, 10, and 15 percent, respectively, for the expected 1955 population. In all instances, production of whole-milk products, fruit, and vegetables would have to be expanded and production of grain products reduced. It would be desirable to produce more meat and poultry in addition to dairy products, fruit, and vegetables, in order to satisfy wants of consumers more fully, if the total volume of food production can be increased. In this case, production of other products such as dry beans and peas and potatoes would need to be reduced substantially.

TABLE 18.—*Food production in 1946 compared with food requirements from domestic production for expected 1955 population with consumption changes which would raise all diets to an adequate level, by major food groups in retail weights, United States*

Food group	1946 food production [1]	Food requirements from domestic production with per capita consumption increased [2]—			Percentage food requirements are of 1946 production with per capita consumption increased [2]—		
		5 percent	10 percent	15 percent	5 percent	10 percent	15 percent
	Million pounds	*Million pounds*	*Million pounds*	*Million pounds*	*Percent*	*Percent*	*Percent*
Dairy products (excluding butter) [3]	86,708	91,120	93,497	95,082	105	108	110
Eggs	7,103	6,202	7,034	7,672	87	99	108
Meat, poultry, and fish	24,394	23,247	26,363	28,759	95	108	118
Fats and oils [4]	9,452	9,776	10,069	10,264	103	107	109
Dry beans, peas, and nuts	2,836	3,424	2,802	2,646	121	99	93
Potatoes and sweetpotatoes	21,545	23,730	19,416	18,337	110	90	85
Citrus fruit and tomatoes	18,362	19,629	20,522	21,413	107	112	117
Leafy, green, and yellow vegetables	18,682	21,922	21,922	21,922	117	117	117
Other vegetables and fruit	34,611	31,019	34,121	37,223	90	99	108
Grain products [5]	42,909	39,574	34,177	30,579	92	80	71
Sugar and sirups	6,158	6,181	6,490	6,799	100	105	110

[1] Estimated retail weight from food production as usually reported by the Bureau of Agricultural Economics in THE NATIONAL FOOD SITUATION by means of average loss factors with the addition of unpublished estimates of supplies from town and city gardens and estimates of minor items.

[2] Computed by multiplying expected 1955 population of 153 million by 1942–45 per capita consumption rates changed as indicated in table 16 to raise all diets to an adequate level and adding estimates for exports and subtracting estimates for imports. Imports and exports are assumed to be the same percentage of total domestic consumption for each food group as in 1935–39 except in the case of sugar. The percentages for net imports are: Dairy

products 0.6, eggs 0.5, meats 2.1, fats and oils 1.7, dry beans and peas 3.1, and leafy, green, and yellow vegetables 0.5, other fruits and vegetables 7.0. Those for net exports are citrus fruit and tomatoes 7.0, and grain products 14.7. It is assumed that net imports of sugar and sirups is 60 percent of total domestic requirements.

[3] Milk equivalent calculated on basis of protein and mineral content. Because of the large exports of dry-milk solids in 1946, exports on this basis were about 9 percent of total production.

[4] Includes butter, bacon, and fat cuts.

[5] Production of all grain except that used for feed and seed converted to grain products equivalent in retail weight.

The pattern of food production that would be required to supply demand as fully as possible in the period ahead, if food habits and preferences do not change, can be indicated at least approximately by assuming that the expected 1955 population will have the same per capita consumption of the various products as in a period of high-level employment.   The year 1946 may be used to represent such a period.   Total food consumption per capita averaged 18 percent higher than in 1935–39 and 7 percent higher than in 1942–45.   Per capita consumption was equal to the estimate which was made in the study referred to earlier (*39, p. 25*) of the per capita consumption that could be expected under full-employment conditions.

Total food requirements for the expected 1955 population, if the 1946 consumption pattern is continued and if the consumption pattern that it was expected would be associated with full employment is achieved, are compared with 1946 production by food groups in table 19.   The total volume of food production would have to be increased only about 2 percent from the 1943–45 level, if imports and exports of food products are the same percentage of total production as in years just before the last war, to make possible this level of per capita consumption.   But substantial changes in output in some food groups would be necessary.

TABLE 19.—*Food production in 1946 compared with requirements from domestic production for the expected 1955 population if the 1946 per capita consumption rates are continued and if the per capita consumption rates associated with high-level employment are realized, and with potential production with improved farming techniques, by major food groups in retail weights, United States*

Food group	1946 food production [1]	Requirements for 1955 population with 1946 consumption rates [2]	Requirements to supply demand with full employment [3]	Production with improved production techniques [4]	Percentage of 1946 food production		
					1946 consumption rates	Demand with full employment	Production with improved techniques
	Million pounds	*Million pounds*	*Million pounds*	*Million pounds*	*Percent*	*Percent*	*Percent*
Dairy products (excluding butter) [5]	86,708	87,295	84,253	94,180	101	97	108
Eggs	7,103	6,851	6,394	6,926	96	90	98
Meat, poultry, and fish	24,394	25,014	25,913	23,843	103	106	98
Fats and oils [6]	9,452	9,626	11,430	12,469	102	120	132
Dry beans, peas, and nuts	2,836	3,262	3,113	4,237	115	110	149
Potatoes and sweetpotatoes	21,545	20,196	18,972	24,659	94	88	114
Citrus fruit and tomatoes	18,362	18,663	19,645	24,371	102	107	133
Leafy, green, and yellow vegetables	18,682	20,399	17,334	18,936	109	93	101
Other vegetables and fruit	34,611	35,572	34,178	38,359	103	100	111
Grain products [7]	42,909	34,221	33,870	36,784	80	81	86
Sugar and sirups	6,158	5,630	7,467	8,644	91	121	140

[1] See footnote 1, table 18.

[2] Total requirements from domestic production computed by multiplying the expected 1955 population of 153 million by the 1946 civilian per capita consumption rates, and adding estimates for exports and subtracting estimates for imports, following the procedure described in footnote 2, table 18.

[3] Total requirements from domestic production computed by multiplying the expected 1955 population of 153 million by the per capita consumption rates that would be associated with high-level employment conditions according to the study of postwar agriculture and employment (*39*), and adding estimates for exports

and subtracting estimates for imports, following the procedure described in footnote 2, table 18.

[4] Estimates of farm production with improved production techniques reported in the study of peacetime production possibilities (*38*), converted to retail weights of food.

[5] Milk equivalent calculated on basis of protein and mineral content. Because of the large exports of dry-milk solids in 1946, exports on this basis were about 9 percent of total production.

[6] Includes butter, bacon, and fat cuts.

[7] Production of all grain except that used for feed and seed converted to grain-products equivalent in retail weight.

Production of grain products, potatoes, and eggs apparently is larger than could be moved into consumption in 1955 even under prosperous business conditions and more than would be required from a dietary standpoint (tables 18 and 19).   Therefore, production of these products may need to be reduced to be in better adjustment with probable demand and dietary needs.   Some of the resources used for their production could be shifted to increase the output of meats, milk, fruit, and vegetables.   In general, the adjustments required to supply probable demand as fully as possible with high-level employment conditions are similar to those that are required to improve diets. This is especially true if the total volume of food production is increased so that it is possible to supply more of the foods people especially want and at the same time supply dietary needs.[21]

Potential production capacity for the various food products in the period ahead also should be considered in deciding what changes in production will be desirable.   For this purpose, the study of peacetime production possibilities, referred to earlier, may be referred to again (table 9, p. 36).   Estimates from this study of production by food groups that would be possible if farmers put into effect improved production methods to the extent they would be profitable and if soil-conserving methods of farming were followed also are shown in table 19.   Total food production would be about 10 percent higher than the average of 1943–45 if this volume of production were realized. Together with the additional food that would be made available if foreign trade returned to prewar levels, this would make possible a 15-percent increase in total consumption per capita.   Therefore, these estimates are comparable with the estimates of production requirements (shown in table 18) if food consumption per capita were increased 15 percent to provide better diets.   The estimates of production with improved production methods are greater than requirements in the case of fats and oils, dry beans and peas, potatoes, and grain products.   But those for livestock products, vegetables, and fruits are less than would be desirable to improve diets as well as to satisfy food preferences as fully as possible.

The shifts in land use required to improve diets and to supply probable demands for foods are in the direction needed for more complete conservation of soil resources.   This is a significant fact, as erosion caused by improper care and use of land has permanently reduced or badly damaged large areas in the United States (*3*).   A shift in production to more livestock products, especially milk and beef cattle, would mean that the acreage of soil-conserving sod crops such as hay and pasture could be increased to replace intertilled crops like corn and soybeans or such close-growing crops as grain in areas where these crops have caused much erosion in the past.   Vegetables and fruit do not use a large part of the total cultivated acreage, and they could be greatly increased in areas where they are now grown, which generally are not subject to erosion.   Adjustments in land use

---

[21] The adjustments indicated by the comparison made in tables 18 and 19 are based on the assumption of the same foreign trade as in 1935–39.   But slow recovery of production in foreign countries may cause imports of fats and oils to be lower than before the war and may make desirable a volume of production in the United States not much lower than at present.   See Hansen and Mighell (*12*).

to conserve soil resources of course would help to make possible a high level of food production on a sustained basis.

ADJUSTMENTS IN FARM PRICES

To improve diets and to supply consumers with more of the foods they want, it will be desirable to maintain prices on a high enough level so that food production will continue to increase. How high prices need to be in order to make further expansion profitable depends upon the changes in cost of items used in production and upon the extent to which more efficient production methods are adopted. The relation between prices received for farm products and prices paid by farmers for commodities, interest, and taxes has averaged nearly 20 percent more favorable for farmers since 1943 than in the 1910–14 period (fig. 9, p. 54). According to the detailed study of production possibilities already referred to, it would be both possible and profitable to increase farm production 10 percent within a few years if more efficient production methods are followed, even though the relation between prices received and prices paid average parity, or the same as in the 1910–14 period (*38*). This means that although prices of farm products should decline considerably our production would probably not be much restricted.

Regardless of the general level of farm prices, some adjustments in price relationships among products can be expected and will be necessary if desirable changes in farm production are to be brought about. Price relationships may need to be modified because of shifts in demand for individual products that take place with changes in population and food preferences or because of shifts in supply that take place with changes in the efficiency with which different products are produced. Because of changes in supply and demand conditions, it cannot be expected that price relationships that were desirable from the standpoint of meeting food needs as fully as possible during the war years will continue to be most desirable in the future (*25*).

The estimates of food requirements from domestic production in 1955 if the 1946 per capita consumption rates are continued and foreign trade returns to prewar levels provide one example of how demand may change in the future (table 19). If prices do not change and incomes per person remain as high as in 1946, the quantities of products indicated apparently would be bought. Total food production would have to be about 2 percent larger than the 1943–45 average to balance demand at these prices, but slightly less than in 1946. It was pointed out in the preceding section that the production pattern would need to be changed to include more livestock products, vegetables, and fruits, and less grain products and potatoes. To bring about such adjustments in production, price relationships for farm products would have to be modified.

Both the total and relative demand for different products may change in other ways. For example, there is the possibility that, because of more widespread knowledge about the beneficial effects on health of consuming more of the foods that are low in cost as sources of nutrients, preferences will change so that consumers will place higher values on the products required to improve diets. In this case somewhat different changes in price relationships would be necessary to bring about the pattern of production that would satisfy demand most fully. The changes in production and prices that would be desirable would depend upon the total volume of production, but in each instance increases in livestock products, fruits, and vegetables in relation to other products would be necessary to supply dietary needs in the kinds of foods that people prefer.

Regardless of how demand for different farm products changes in the future, some adjustments in price relationships probably will be desirable because of shifts in supply that result from changes in the efficiency with which individual products can be produced. The estimates of production changes that are possible if improved farming techniques are followed to the extent they would be profitable with assumed prices for products provide one example of how the supply of farm products may change in the period ahead (table 9).

The possibilities of increasing the efficiency with which different products are produced can be expected to differ. For example, if it is correct that opportunities for introducing more efficient production methods are greater for livestock than for crop products, somewhat less favorable prices for livestock in relation to crop products than in the past would be required to obtain the same volume of output of each in the future. But if production of livestock products needs to be expanded more than that of other products, it still may be true that prices need to favor livestock.

EFFECTS OF MORE EFFICIENT PRODUCTION METHODS

Total demand for food products in the future may not be large enough to make profitable an expansion in farm production to the extent possible or necessary to provide better diets with the kinds of food people prefer. But if costs of food products can be reduced by widespread adoption of more efficient farming methods or more efficient processing and distribution methods, a larger quantity of food could be bought by consumers without increasing their expenditures for food. It would be especially desirable to reduce the production costs of the products that are required to improve diets, because the consumption changes would be more quickly achieved in that way. Even though food preferences do not change, people then would be likely to buy more of the products that are required for better diets.

Production per farm worker and crop production per acre could be increased nearly 20 percent within a few years, according to the study of production possibilities with improved farming methods (*38, p. 5*). Increased yields per acre would come mainly from greater use of lime and fertilizer but also from improved plant varieties and cultural practices. Higher crop yields would increase the productivity of farm workers because labor requirements would not increase proportionately. But greater mechanization on farms would be the main influence in increasing the productivity of farm workers. Employment of additional resources, such as fertilizer and machinery, in farm production would be partly responsible for the 10-percent increase in total food production which was estimated as possible, but productivity per unit of resources employed in agriculture probably would be increased nearly 10 percent.

Detailed information about how the cost of producing different products may be affected by more efficient production methods is not available. There has been more rapid progress in increasing efficiency in crop than in livestock production in the past (table 3).   But the possibilities of introducing improved methods in livestock production are great.   This is especially true in the case of milk, which uses relatively large amounts of labor as compared with other products. In fact, all the products required in larger quantities to improve diets as well as to satisfy food preferences—livestock, vegetables, and fruits—use relatively large amounts of farm labor as compared with grains, oil-bearing crops, dry beans and peas, and potatoes, all of which may need to be reduced.

Two conditions will be necessary to bring about rapid improvement in the efficiency of farm production.   The first is an expanding market for farm products and the second is opportunity for other work for those not needed in agriculture.   Most of the improved farming methods do not lower cash expenditures and may even involve some additional expenditures for machinery and materials.   They do make possible a larger output with the same labor and land, but unless the additional output can be sold without causing prices of farm products to decline, the additional expenditures may exceed the value of the additional output.   Some expansion in total farm output probably will take place through the adoption of improved farming methods even if farm prices decline.   But expansion will come about most rapidly if demand for farm products increases so that a larger total output can be sold without reducing farm prices.   In this case, the new methods that increase output per farm would be highly profitable.

As farm workers are largely self-employed, unit costs of production usually cannot be reduced by substituting mechanical methods for hand labor to produce the same volume of output.   But it is possible that costs could be reduced without increasing total output if the labor displaced by mechanical methods can find employment elsewhere. Employment conditions like those that have prevailed in recent years would help to encourage the shift of farm workers into other occupations and would reduce the use of labor resources in agriculture.

EFFECTS ON FARM INCOMES

As future expansion in farm production depends mainly upon its profitableness, the conditions under which an expansion would result in a larger net farm income should be considered.   How income would be affected by expanding production depends upon the effects of a larger output on the cost per unit of product and on the level of farm prices.   It is apparent from the previous discussion that lower costs per unit of product would be possible if farm production is increased by further adoption of improved methods such as those that have been responsible in the past for reducing the physical costs per unit of product.

The information that is available about the effects of a larger output on farm prices is not conclusive, but one source states that "consumer demand for many products—and possibly the composite demand for foods as a whole—is inelastic in the sense that consumers will spend more total money for a small supply than a large one" (*10, pp. 15 and 16*).   This means that prices would decline by a greater percentage than total output is increased.   Although demand for all farm products considered together may be inelastic, it is known that demand for certain products—such as livestock, vegetables, and fruit—is much more elastic than for others—such as grain, dry beans and peas, and potatoes (7, pp. 61 and 62). Also, elasticity of demand for food products apparently is greatest in the case of people whose incomes are relatively low. Therefore the effects of increasing the total volume of production on the level of farm prices in the future will depend not only on the changes in the national income or total demand but also upon the products that are produced in larger quantities and the changes in the distribution of income among consumers.

Demand for farm products would need to be relatively elastic to make an expansion in farm production result in a larger net income to farm operators even though the larger output is achieved by more widespread application of farming methods that do not increase the production costs. For example, if farm production were increased 10

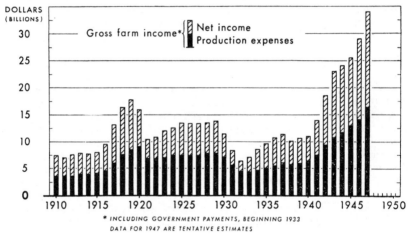

FIGURE 10.—Gross farm income: net income and production expenses of farm operators, United States, 1910–47.

percent from the 1943–45 average level without any additional costs, it would be necessary that farm prices should not decline by more than 10 percent if net farm income is to remain the same. On the other hand, if demand should increase during the period when production is being expanded, so that prices decline less than 10 percent, the net income from agriculture would be increased.

Net income of farm operators has been relatively high in recent years as the result of increased demand for farm products for export and domestic use (fig. 10). But what would be the effect on income if foreign trade should return to the prewar level and food production be further expanded by more widespread application of the more efficient farming methods? A 10-percent increase in farm production, together with exports and imports of food products averaging the same percentage of total production as in 1935–39, would make possible a per capita consumption 15 percent higher than in 1943–45 and 8 percent higher than in 1946 for the expected 1955 population (table 14). Demand for farm products for domestic use would have to be considerably larger than in 1943–45 before this higher level of consumption could be achieved, with only a 10-percent decline in prices. But if this were possible, the volume of production that would be available could be disposed of without reducing gross or net farm income. If production expenses of farm operators could be reduced 10 percent, the net farm income of farm operators would be increased 7 percent.

These computations show that an expansion in domestic demand for farm products will be necessary if income of farmers on a level something like that in recent years is to be maintained. If demand is not increased and if farm prices decline as much as 30 percent as total production is increased 10 percent, net income would be reduced about 50 percent. But net income would be reduced only about 40 percent if production costs were reduced 10 percent.

It still would be possible to maintain incomes of those engaged in farming on the present level if the number of workers in agriculture could be reduced substantially by utilizing more labor-saving methods. The general public would benefit, for the lower prices would make possible a larger volume of consumption.

Balancing Supply and Demand

Earnings of domestic consumers and purchases for export and foreign relief have continued to be high since the end of the war. Total demand for food from the United States has remained so great that nearly everything produced has sold at prices relatively profitable to producers. But this general situation may change, especially if the per capita supply of food for domestic consumption is increased. The changes in production and consumption of food products that have been described as desirable in the future, under defined conditions with respect to the total food-production capacity, could be achieved most readily if domestic demand should change, as indicated by the additional expenditures for food products (table 17). But failure of demand to change in this way would not make such changes any less desirable from the standpoint of utilizing resources as fully and efficiently as possible.

If incomes and expenditures of consumers for food decline from recent levels, however, farm incomes also would be reduced. In such a situation it would be desirable to know what measures could be taken to help maintain incomes of farmers adequately and at the same time help to bring about the adjustments in production and consumption that are desirable from a national standpoint.

If total demand for farm products is inelastic in the sense that a small output will have a greater market value than a larger one, it would be possible to increase gross farm income by reducing total output. But this would mean that farm resources would not be fully utilized and that food needs would not be met as fully as possible. Moreover, it would be difficult if not impossible to achieve an over-all reduction in farm production except over a long period because it usually is most profitable for individual farmers to utilize their resources fully and maintain or expand production regardless of changes in farm prices. Relatively low farm prices would eventually cause resources, especially labor, to be shifted from agriculture to other uses and thus cause farm production to be reduced, but this would take place only over a period of several years and then only if other employment were available. Even if a reduction in farm production were possible within a short period, it would be desirable from a national standpoint only if the resources not required in agriculture could be shifted to other uses where the value of their output would be greater.

The development and application of more efficient methods of production and distribution which reduce costs per unit of product would make profitable a larger volume of farm production even though prices decline. Lower prices of course would make possible a larger volume of food consumption without increasing total expenditures. But, as pointed out above, most improved farming methods increase output per farm with the same land and labor and do not greatly reduce cash costs of operation. Farm costs of production cannot be reduced very much by substituting mechanical methods for hand labor unless the displaced labor can find other employment.

More efficient production methods can be used to produce a larger total output with the same resources and in this way reduce unit costs, but it is necessary that market outlets at no great reduction in prices be available for the additional output to prevent net incomes of farmers from declining.

It is apparent that total demand for food products must be stabilized on a relatively high level to achieve a high level of food consumption per capita and to assure adequate incomes to farmers. A continuation of business conditions like those of recent years, for example, would mean that total demand for domestic consumption would be great enough so that with some gradual reduction in costs of producing and distributing food products the present volume of food production could be marketed at prices profitable to producers. On the other hand, if total demand should decline greatly within a short period, it would be impossible to reduce total production or production costs enough to prevent farm incomes from declining. Under such conditions it would be desirable to utilize special programs to maintain and expand the total demand for food products (*28, 29, 30*). But any programs that are put into operation to expand demand or to help maintain farm incomes on an adequate level should be designed so that they help to achieve the adjustments in production and consumption that have been described as necessary to make full and efficient use of available food-production resources.

THE MEANING OF IT ALL

From the beginning of World War I to the beginning of World War II, food production in the United States increased about one-third. This took place gradually at about the same rate as growth in total population, or 1 percent annually. From 1935–39 to 1946, food production increased another one-third at the more rapid average rate of about 3 percent annually. Food production per capita has averaged 27 percent higher in the last few years than it did before the war. Although much more food was exported and less was imported, consumption per capita was 10 percent higher in 1942–45 and 18 percent higher in 1946 than it was in 1935–39. But in the years ahead food consumption per capita can average 15 percent higher than it did during the war years or 8 percent higher than it did in 1946 if the prewar rate of increase in production, about the same as population growth, is resumed and exports and imports of food products are the same percentage of total production as in the prewar period. Even though the total volume of food production does not rise from the wartime level, an increase of 5 percent in consumption per capita from the wartime average, or only slightly lower than the level in 1946, would be possible for the expected 1955 population.

The total volume of food production in the next few years will depend in part upon changes in demand for food products. But output probably will not be reduced even though farm prices decline and probably will be increased if farm prices remain the same, or increase. Both the long-term and wartime increases in farm production have been achieved mainly by more widespread application of improved production methods which raised output per acre and per worker. The total acreage of harvested cropland increased about 10 percent from 1910 to 1920, but it has not changed so very much since then. Total employment of farm workers decreased 10 percent from 1910 to 1940 and an additional 8 percent during the recent war. More machinery, fertilizer, and other resources have been used to increase the productivity of land and labor, but total output per unit of all resources employed in agriculture has increased, especially in recent years.

Employment of resources in agriculture would not be reduced even though farm prices should decrease because it still would be profitable for individual farmers to utilize their resources fully. The more efficient production methods that have been adopted undoubtedly will be continued because they will be profitable even with lower farm prices. But new developments in farm technology will be applied most rapidly in the future if farm prices remain relatively high.

The expansion in the productive capacity of agriculture makes it possible to supply food needs and wants more fully than ever before. Many people still have diets that are nutritionally inadequate, and most people do not receive all of certain kinds of food they would like. Per capita consumption of food nutrients (protein, minerals, and vitamins) would have to be increased substantially from the 1942 level if the diets of all people that are below the recommended allowances of the National Research Council were brought up to this level and if those that consumed more continue to do so. Dietary deficiencies are greatest among people with low incomes, but not all those with high incomes have adequate diets. It would be possible to provide market outlet for all the food products that can be produced in the near future by changing the national consumption pattern to include more of the products that people want and would buy in larger quantities if they had enough income. For example, about 30 percent more food would have been consumed in 1942 if food consumption by all people in the United States had averaged the same as it did for those in families that had annual incomes of $3,000 or more.

On the other hand, the total food supply measured in terms of food nutrients could be increased greatly by changing the national pattern of food production to include more of the products that provide relatively large outputs of nutrients per unit of resources. For example, 7 to 10 times as much food energy is obtained from farm land and labor used to produce grain products, potatoes, and certain vegetables as from the same resources when used to produce livestock products.

Milk is the lowest cost source of protein among livestock products, but some food crops, such as dry beans and peas, grain products, and potatoes, provide three to four times as much protein as does milk per unit of farm resources. Whole-grain products, dry beans, and peas and whole-milk products are the most efficient sources of calcium and riboflavin. Citrus fruit and certain vegetables are the lowest cost sources of vitamins A and C; thiamine and niacin can be obtained most efficiently from cereals, dry beans and peas, potatoes, and certain other vegetables. Because of these differences, the number of people that can be supplied with adequate diets from available resources depends upon the diet that is consumed. For example, 200 million people could be supplied with a low-cost diet with the present cropland area and yields per acre equal to those of wartime but only 140 million with a relatively high-cost diet. To support 200 million people with adequate diets, of course, would require shifts in consumption to more of the foods that do not satisfy tastes or preferences very well.

It would be possible to supply the additional nutrients required to improve diets without employing more resources or using more efficient production methods by changing the pattern of production and consumption to include more of the products that provide larger outputs of nutrients per unit of resources. But this would require changes in consumption that people would not like to make and that are not necessary as long as the total food supply for domestic use can be increased. The extent to which tastes and preferences for foods can be satisfied and at the same time additional needs for nutrients to improve diets be supplied will depend upon the extent to which food consumption per capita can be increased, and that, in turn, will depend upon the total volume of food production.

Future changes in the total volume of food production cannot be predicted exactly, but three possibilities can be considered. They are no change, a 5-percent increase, and a 10-percent increase from the wartime volume of production. These changes, together with the additional food that would be available if exports and imports of food were to average the same percentage of total food production as in the 1935–39 period, would make possible increases in food consumption per capita from the 1943–45 wartime average of 5 percent, 10 percent, and 15 percent, respectively, for the expected 1955 population. Needs for additional nutrients could be met with only a 5-percent increase in per capita consumption, but it then would be necessary to reduce consumption of meat, eggs, and certain vegetables and fruit, to make possible the necessary increases in whole-milk products, other vegetables and fruit, cereals, dry beans and peas, and potatoes, which are sources of nutrients with lower costs.

But if per capita consumption can be increased 10 or 15 percent, it would be possible to improve diets with more of the products that people especially prefer in larger quantities, such as meat, eggs, dairy products, and certain vegetables and fruits. Consumption of cereals, dry beans and peas, and some other products would be reduced, and average consumption would become more like that of people in the high-income groups.

Farm production was adjusted to meet changes in food needs that arose during the war, but it must be modified in the period ahead if food requirements for better nutrition and for probable demand are to be met as fully as possible. Shifts in production that will be required if diets are to be improved will differ, depending upon the extent to which the total volume of food production is increased. But for all the possibilities considered, increases in whole-milk products, citrus fruit and tomatoes, and leafy, green, and yellow vegetables will be necessary. Changes in production of most products also will be necessary to supply probable demand more fully. Changes in production to improve nutrition and to meet demand will be most alike if total consumption can be increased so as to provide better diets with products that also satisfy tastes and preferences. Some modification from recent price relationships for farm products will be necessary if these adjustments in farm production are to be brought about.

Domestic demand for food will have to remain on a high level to provide market outlets for products in the quantities that can be produced with available resources. But even if total demand is not large enough to maintain prices of farm products that will be as profitable as in recent years, it still will be desirable to achieve the adjustments in production and consumption that have been described as necessary to make full and efficient use of resources. Of course, it also will be desirable to maintain incomes of food producers on an adequate level. Reduction in total output would result in larger total income to farmers, if total demand for farm products is so inelastic that a smaller output will have a larger total value than a larger output. But individual farmers will not find it to their advantage to reduce output, because most of their costs will remain fixed. Moreover, expansion in total production will be highly desirable from a national standpoint.

Regardless of how demand may change, more efficient methods of producing and distributing food products should be pushed forward as rapidly as possible because they would make profitable a larger volume of production even if prices decline. They would increase the purchasing power of consumers and make possible a larger volume of consumption with the same expenditures for food. Of course, public programs that influence production and consumption of food products can be arranged so that they help to bring about desirable adjustments.

LITERATURE CITED

(1) ATKINSON, L. J., and KLEIN, J. W.
   1946. FEED CONSUMPTION AND PRODUCTION OF PORK AND LARD. U. S. Dept. Agr. Tech. Bul. 917, 21 pp., illus.
(2) BEESON, K. C.
   1941. THE MINERAL COMPOSITION OF CROPS WITH PARTICULAR REFERENCE TO THE SOILS IN WHICH THEY WERE GROWN. U. S. Dept. Agr. Misc. Pub. 369, 164 pp., illus.
(3) BENNETT, H. H.
   1946. OUR AMERICAN LAND—THE STORY OF ITS ABUSE AND ITS CONSERVATION. U. S. Dept. Agr. Misc. Pub. 596, 31 pp., illus.
(4) CLARK, FAITH, FRIEND, BERTA, and BURK, M. C.
   1947. NUTRITIVE VALUE OF THE PER CAPITA FOOD SUPPLY, 1909–45. U. S. Dept. Agr. Misc. Pub. 616, 36 pp., illus.
(5) COCHRANE, W. W.
   1945. HIGH LEVEL FOOD CONSUMPTION IN THE UNITED STATES. U. S. Dept. Agr. Misc. Pub, 581, 48 pp., illus.
(6) COOPER, MARTIN R., BARTON, G. T., and BRODELL, A. P.
   1947. PROGRESS IN FARM MECHANIZATION. U. S. Dept. Agr. Misc. Pub. 630, 101 pp., illus.

(7) EZEKIEL, MORDECAI, and BEAN, L. H.
    1933. ECONOMIC BASIS FOR THE AGRICULTURAL ADJUSTMENT ACT. U. S.
        Dept. Agr., 67 pp., illus.
(8) FOOD AND AGRICULTURE ORGANIZATION OF THE UNITED NATIONS.
    1946. WORLD FOOD SURVEY. 39 pp., illus., Washington, D. C.
(9) GILBERT, S. J.
    1945. WISCONSIN DAIRY PRODUCTION, UTILIZATION, AND RELATED DATA.
        Wis. Dept. Agr. Bul. 250, pp. 19–27. Madison.
(10) GOLD, N. L., HOFFMAN, A. C., and WAUGH, F. V.
    1940. ECONOMIC ANALYSIS OF THE FOOD STAMP PLAN. U. S. Dept. Agr.
        Special Report, 98 pp., illus.
(11) HANSEN, A. C., and CORNFIELD, J.
    1942. SPENDING AND SAVING OF THE NATION'S FAMILIES IN WARTIME.
        U. S. Bur. Labor Statis. Bul. 723, 22 pp., illus.
(12) HANSEN, P. L., and MIGHELL, R. L.
    1947. OIL CROPS IN AMERICAN FARMING. U. S. Dept. Agr. Tech. Bul.
        940, 55 pp., illus.
(13) JENSEN, EINAR, KLEIN, JOHN W., RAUCHENSTEIN, EMIL, WOODWARD,
        T. E., and SMITH, R. H.
    1942. INPUT-OUTPUT RELATIONSHIPS IN MILK PRODUCTION. U. S. Dept.
        Agr. Tech. Bul. 815, 88 pp., illus.
(14) KLING, WILLIAM
    1943. FOOD WASTE IN DISTRIBUTION AND USE. Jour. Farm Econ.
        25:848–859.
(15) MAYNARD, L. A.
    1947. DEFICIENCIES IN THE UNITED STATES DIET AND MEANS OF MEETING
        THEM. Jour. Farm Econ. 29:321–323.
(16) ―――
    1944. FOOD PRODUCTION FOR BETTER HEALTH AND LONGER LIFE. Con-
        ference . . . under the sponsorship of the Research Labora-
        tory of the Children's Fund of Michigan. Proc. (Implications
        of Nutrition and Public Health in the Postwar Period) pp. 5–19.
        Detroit.
(17) ―――
    1946. THE ROLE AND EFFICIENCY OF ANIMALS IN UTILIZING FEED TO
        PRODUCE HUMAN FOOD. Jour. Nutrition 32: 345–361.
(18) MENDERSHAUSEN, HORST.
    1946. CHANGES IN INCOME DISTRIBUTION DURING THE GREAT DEPRESSION.
        Nat'l Bur. Econ. Res. Inc. Conf. on Income and Wealth,
        Studies. v. 7, 173 pp., illus. New York.
(19) NATIONAL PLANNING ASSOCIATION.
    1945. A FOOD AND NUTRITION PROGRAM FOR THE NATION. Nat'l Planning
        Assoc. Planning Pam. 46, 35 pp.
(20) NATIONAL RESEARCH COUNCIL.
    1945. RECOMMENDED DIETARY ALLOWANCES. Nat'l Res. Council. Reprint
        and Cir. Ser. 122, revised. 6 pp.
(21) ―――
    1943. INADEQUATE DIETS AND NUTRITIONAL DEFICIENCIES IN THE UNITED
        STATES. Nat'l Res. Council. Number 109. 56 pp.
(22) NELSON, A. G.
    1945. RELATION OF FEED CONSUMED TO FOOD PRODUCTS PRODUCED BY
        FATTENING CATTLE. U. S. Dept. Agr. Tech. Bul. 900, 36 pp.,
        illus.
(23) PEARL, RAYMOND.
    1920. THE NATION'S FOOD. 274 pp., illus. Philadelphia, Pa.
(24) SCHULTZ, T. W.
    1945. AGRICULTURE IN AN UNSTABLE ECONOMY. 299 pp., illus. New
        York, N. Y.
(25) ―――
    1943. FARM PRICES FOR FOOD PRODUCTION. Iowa State Col. Wartime
        Farm and Food Policy Pam. 2, 43 pp. Ames.
(26) SCHICKELE, RAINER
    1947. NATIONAL FOOD POLICY AND SURPLUS AGRICULTURAL PRODUCTION.
        Jour. Farm Econ. 29: 867–888

(27) SHERMAN, H. C.
    1944. PRINCIPLES OF NUTRITION AND NUTRITIVE VALUE OF FOODS. U. S.
        Dept. Agr. Misc. Pub. 546, 40 pp.
(28) SOUTHWORTH, H. M.
    1945. THE ECONOMICS OF PUBLIC MEASURES TO SUBSIDIZE FOOD CONSUMP-
        TION. Jour. Farm Econ. 27: 38–67.
(29) —————— and KLAYMAN, M. I.
    1941. THE SCHOOL LUNCH PROGRAM AND AGRICULTURAL SURPLUS DISPOSAL.
        U. S. Dept. Agr. Misc. Pub. 467, 66 pp., illus.
(30) STIEBELING, H. K., FARIOLETTI, MARIUS, WAUGH, F. V., and CAVIN, J. P.
    1939. BETTER NUTRITION AS A NATIONAL GOAL. U. S. Dept. Agr. Yearbook
        Agr. (Food and Life) 1939: 380–405.
(31) —————— and CLARK, FAITH.
    1939. PLANNING FOR GOOD NUTRITION. U. S. Dept. Agr. Yearbook Agr.
        (Food and Life) 1939: 321–341.
(32) TOLLEY, H. R.
    1945. AGRICULTURAL ADJUSTMENT AND NUTRITION. In SCHULTZ, T. W.,
        ed. FOOD FOR THE WORLD, pp. 164–177. Chicago.
(33) UNITED STATES BUREAU OF AGRICULTURAL ECONOMICS.
    1945. PRICE SPREADS BETWEEN FARMERS AND CONSUMERS FOR FOOD
        PRODUCTS, 1913–44. U. S. Dept. Agr. Misc. Pub. 576, 290 pp., illus.
(34) UNITED STATES BUREAU OF HUMAN NUTRITION AND HOME ECONOMICS.
    1944. FAMILY FOOD CONSUMPTION IN THE UNITED STATES, SPRING 1942.
        U. S. Dept. Agr. Misc. Pub. 550, 157 pp.
(35)——————
    1945. TABLES OF FOOD COMPOSITION IN TERMS OF ELEVEN NUTRIENTS.
        U. S. Dept. Agr. Misc. Pub. 572, 30 pp.
(36) ——————
    1948. HELPING FAMILIES PLAN FOOD BUDGETS. U. S. Dept. Agr. Misc.
        Pub. (In Press.)
(37) UNITED STATES BUREAU OF LABOR STATISTICS.
    1945. FAMILY SPENDING AND SAVING IN WARTIME. U. S. Dept. Labor
        Bul. 822, 218 pp., illus.
(38) UNITED STATES DEPARTMENT OF AGRICULTURE.
    1945. PEACETIME ADJUSTMENTS IN FARMING. POSSIBILITIES UNDER PROS-
        PERITY CONDITIONS. U. S. Dept. Agr. Misc. Pub. 595, 52 pp.,
        illus.
(39) ——————
    1945. WHAT PEACE CAN MEAN TO AMERICAN FARMERS. POST-WAR AGRI-
        CULTURE AND EMPLOYMENT. U. S. Dept. Agr. Misc. Pub. 562,
        28 pp.

ADDITIONAL TABLES

TABLE 20.—*Average outputs of farm products, food at retail, and food nutrients per acre of feed crops used to produce specified livestock products* [1]

Farm product and food use	Farm products	Food at retail	Number of days a moderately active man can be supplied with a daily allowance of each of the food nutrients [2]										
			Food energy	Protein	Fat	Calcium	Iron	Vitamin A	Thiamine	Ascorbic acid	Riboflavin	Niacin	Average of 10 nutrients
	Pounds	Pounds	Days	Days	Days	Days	Days	Days	Days	Days	Days	Days	Days
Dairy products:													
Milk, whole	1,065	1,038	108	236	245	696	26	150	111	83	405	35	210
Evaporated milk	1,065	498	105	226	238	686	33	181	73	33	406	30	201
Butter	1,065	52	58	2	257	5	4	157	0	0	1	2	49
Cheese, American	1,065	106	63	164	206	523	23	167	14	0	121	6	129
All dairy products [3]	1,065	590	87	148	246	442	19	156	62	46	244	21	147
Dairy enterprise [4]			68	125	196	306	34	107	53	32	179	27	113
Poultry:													
Chicken enterprise [5]	263		49	186	140	50	186	153	66	12	118	100	106
Eggs	256	255	54	188	158	70	232	234	80	0	172	5	119
Chickens	287	225	40	180	105	12	99	0	39	34	15	279	80
Broilers	205	253	45	201	117	14	111	0	44	38	17	312	90
Turkeys		187	50	163	152	8	146	0	36	30	14	253	85
Hogs:													
Pork and lard	339	240	183	129	765	7	129	0	704	0	71	365	236
Pork		189	114	129	458	7	129	0	704	0	71	365	185
Lard		51	69	0	307	0	0	0		0	0	0	51
Cattle:													
All beef cattle	165	81	27	77	88	4	67	0	32	0	34	171	50
Fattening cattle	165	81	27	77	88	4	67	0	32	0	34	171	50

Sheep:												
All sheep	61	30	11	23	39	2	26	0	0	34	18	35	19
Fattening lambs	149	72	26	57	94	4	23	0	0	84	43	85	42

[1] Average outputs are for the land actually used to produce the feed crops fed to each class of livestock, using 1941–45 average crop yields. To convert all land to cropland equivalent, the feed obtained from pasture is assumed to have a yield equal to all tame hay. The outputs shown do not include an allowance for byproducts which indirectly are sources of food or for the nonfood byproducts. The farm value of these byproducts expressed as percentages of the total farm value of all the products derived from the farm product in the 1943–45 period are as follows: milk for butter—10, milk for cheese—4, beef cattle—17, sheep—29, and hogs—1.

[2] Computed by dividing the nutrient content of the food at retail by daily allowances of food nutrients for a moderately active man, as recommended by the National Research Council.

[3] All milk used for dairy products as in the 1943–45 period.

[4] Includes cull cows, veal calves, and all milk used, as in the 1943–45 period.

[5] Includes chickens and eggs in the combination they were produced in the 1943–45 period.

TABLE 21.—*Average outputs of farm products, food at retail, and food nutrients per acre of land used to produce specified food crops* [1]

Farm product and food use	Farm products	Food at retail	Number of days a moderately active man can be supplied with a daily allowance of each of the food nutrients [2]										
			Food energy	Protein	Fat	Calcium	Iron	Vitamin A	Thiamine	Ascorbic acid	Riboflavin	Niacin	Average of 10 nutrients
	Pounds	Pounds	Days	Days	Days	Days	Days	Days	Days	Days	Days	Days	Days
Grain:													
Barley, pearl barley	1,166	642	347	341	39	59	486	0	235	0	119	604	223
Buckwheat, flour	870	487	261	198	32	31	183	0	458	0	87	309	156
Corn, yellow corn meal	1,837	1,312	725	773	294	136	1,344	611	1,784	0	492	813	697
Corn, cornflakes	1,837	689	375	354	29	39	258	0	330	0	135	330	185
Oats, oatmeal	1,040	428	257	395	191	132	842	0	711	0	135	148	281
Rice, white	2,007	1,325	704	654	24	68	353	0	212	0	79	557	265
Rice, brown	2,007	1,585	855	772	163	351	3,303	0	1,406	0	174	2,188	921
Rye, light flour	706	537	291	309	30	55	264	0	244	0	84	147	142
Rye, whole flour	706	668	364	485	69	231	1,212	0	948	0	313	352	397
Wheat, white flour	1,062	754	405	527	41	81	189	0	151	0	57	176	163
Wheat, whole flour	1,062	1,041	566	877	126	225	1,500	0	1,756	0	291	1,756	710
Other staple food crops:													
Beans, dry edible	889	782	414	1,116	71	656	3,050	0	1,413	83	419	500	772
Peas, split peas	1,322	1,124	602	1,785	67	465	2,548	378	2,953	141	731	1,034	1,070
Potatoes, Irish	8,328	7,445	806	812	43	391	1,674	104	1,985	6,404	561	2,183	1,496
Sweetpotatoes	4,912	4,224	687	421	151	620	949	25,369	1,041	4,846	486	789	3,536
Peanuts, peanut butter	668	381	355	643	1,099	160	272	0	225	0	136	1,862	475
Soybeans, whole edible	1,092	983	521	2,224	1,078	1,267	2,973	96	3,394	0	688	618	1,286
Sugar beets, gran. sugar	24,800	3,646	2,199	0	0	0	145	0	0	0	0	0	234
Sugarcane, gran. sugar	41,200	3,098	1,868	0	0	0	137	.	0	0	0	0	200
Sugar beets, brn. sugar	24,800	3,894	2,249	0	0	1,673	3,823	0	0	0	0	0	774
Sugarcane, brn. sugar	41,200	3,317	1,923	0	0	1,442	3,262	0	0	0	0	0	663

Oil-bearing crops:										
Cottonseed	446	64	87	0	389	0	0	0	0	0	48
Peanuts	668	183	250	0	1,107	0	0	0	0	0	136
Soybeans	1,092	154	210	0	932	0	0	0	0	0	114

¹ Average yields in 1941–45 period. The outputs shown do not include an allowance for the value of byproducts or joint products such as feeds which indirectly are a source of food and for the non-food products. The farm value of these byproducts and joint products expressed as percentages of the total farm value of all the products derived from the farm product in the 1943–45 period are as follows: Corn for cornflakes—63, corn for corn meal—20, wheat for white flour—25, wheat for whole-wheat flour—7, wheat for macaroni—60, rice—24, sugar beets for sugar—7, sugarcane for sugar—4, cotton for oil—88, peanuts for oil—31, and soybeans for oil—58.

² Computed by dividing the nutrient content of the food at retail by daily allowances of food nutrients for a moderately active man, as recommended by the National Research Council.

TABLE 22.—*Average outputs of farm products, food at retail, and food nutrients per acre of land used to produce specified vegetables* [1]

Farm product and food use	Farm products	Food at retail	Number of days a moderately active man can be supplied with a daily allowance of each of the food nutrients [2]										
			Food energy	Protein	Fat	Calcium	Iron	Vitamin A	Thiamine	Ascorbic acid	Riboflavin	Niacin	Average of 10 nutrients
	Pounds	*Pounds*	*Days*	*Days*	*Days*	*Days*	*Days*	*Days*	*Days*	*Days*	*Days*	*Days*	*Days*
Fresh vegetables:													
Asparagus	2,448	2,227	67	239	21	198	575	1,528	802	3,356	657	579	802
Beans, lima	2,112	1,943	154	378	39	279	680	202	583	1,503	253	220	429
Beans, snap	2,700	2,403	138	336	26	799	901	1,230	513	2,531	493	401	737
Beets	9,516	8,565	442	661	34	985	2,426	137	628	3,882	728	799	1,072
Cabbage	13,840	11,764	373	773	110	2,235	1,662	635	1,804	27,135	1,236	706	3,667
Cantaloups	6,660	5,661	90	105	30	255	424	8,254	452	5,208	227	642	1,569
Carrots	16,350	14,715	878	1,009	235	2,869	3,924	141,265	2,649	4,709	1,914	1,962	16,141
Cauliflower	10,804	9,291	195	650	50	523	1,703	371	1,301	17,468	1,022	743	2,403
Celery	27,300	24,570	516	1,299	197	4,392	2,867		1,474	6,552	1,474	1,474	2,024
Cucumbers	5,136	4,417	68	139	18	177	368	0	353	1,590	619	147	348
Eggplant	7,590	6,603	245	406	71	487	880	132	1,189	1,673	726	1,409	722
Kale	6,876	5,570	267	899	127	4,560	2,971	24,450	1,300	24,877	2,813	891	6,316
Lettuce	10,710	8,675	165	471	70	748	1,157	2,967	1,157	2,776	911	289	1,071
Onions	12,900	11,094	769	951	133	1,900	1,942	466	1,110	5,621	555	444	1,389
Peas, green	2,610	2,479	170	486	27	140	806	690	1,190	1,786	459	694	645
Peppers, green	5,650	5,086	190	334	55	267	635	2,451	916	30,984	433	474	3,674
Spinach	3,816	3,091	95	380	45	1,163	2,885	21,661	907	9,025	1,391	536	3,809
Sweet corn	3,491	3,002	187	274	84	60	226	409	541	801	360	480	3,342
Tomatoes	6,201	4,650	141	266	74	255	930	4,074	744	5,767	372	775	1,340
Watermelons	6,975	6,068	132	87	33	114	202	1,505	404	1,052	334	162	402

Canned vegetables:													
Asparagus	2,360	1,615	51	168	30	184	605	888	312	1,442	315	398	439
Beans, green lima	1,116	1,590	174	393	30	245	1,020	188	169	763	175	233	339
Beans, snap	3,340	4,523	132	291	0	695	2,411	1,701	422	1,086	498	452	769
Beets	14,120	4,688	275	301		398	1,055	75	156	1,313	305	157	404
Cabbage for kraut	16,840	12,967	389	926	155	3,387	2,485	130	1,210	13,832	5,900	865	2,928
Peas, green	1,790	2,551	265	561	62	364	1,742	1,260	816	1,326	332	697	742
Spinach	4,580	4,946	185	735	118	2,528	3,009	30,500	296	4,353	940	462	4,307
Sweet corn	4,680	1,756	204	229	54	40	336	323	129	561	185	445	251
Tomatoes	10,220	4,476	144	288	53	279	1,007	4,271	686	4,476	336	954	1,249

¹ Average yields in 1936–45 period.
² Computed by dividing the nutrient content of the food at retail by daily allowances of food nutrients for a moderately active man, as recommended by the National Research Council.

TABLE 23.—*Average outputs of farm products, food at retail, and food nutrients per acre of land used to produce fruits* [1]

| Farm product and food use | Farm products | Food at retail | Number of days a moderately active man can be supplied with a daily allowance of each of the food nutrients [2] | | | | | | | | | | |
			Food energy	Protein	Fat	Calcium	Iron	Vitamin A	Thiamine	Ascorbic acid	Riboflavin	Niacin	Average of 10 nutrients
	Pounds	*Pounds*	*Days*	*Days*	*Days*	*Days*	*Days*	*Days*	*Days*	*Days*	*Days*	*Days*	*Days*
Fresh fruit:													
Apples	5,184	4,666	401	80	100	140	467	336	467	1,120	186	311	361
Apricots	6,192	5,635	453	346	30	479	986	13,444	489	1,127	479	1,202	1,904
Avocados	2,176	1,980	595	164	2,371	84	330	384	555	1,426	505	488	690
Grapefruit	21,390	20,320	901	435	163	1,295	1,524	284	1,490	32,784	610	813	4,030
Grapes	8,009	7,208	778	360	173	676	1,562	476	1,153	1,634	432	913	816
Lemons	18,240	17,328	710	619	393	845	433	0	1,502	29,342	86	462	3,439
Limes	2,640	2,508	154	100	10	150	63	0	267	3,143	25	84	400
Oranges	14,800	14,060	769	582	131	1,898	1,523	1,743	2,343	30,370	562	750	4,067
Peaches	5,760	5,126	349	146	27	205	1,025	3,619	273	2,119	487	1,230	948
Pears	8,700	7,830	684	291	157	480	718	141	417	1,670	626	261	544
Plums	5,700	4,984	402	214	60	455	914	1,505	2,093	1,329	324	797	809
Blueberries	916	888	92	34	32	81	267	229	71	877	134	77	189
Strawberries	2,241	2,017	120	101	70	308	588	101	175	7,019	292	175	895
Dried fruit:													
Apples, nuggets	5,184	518	306	47	31	71	804	0	83	346	30	79	186
Apricots	6,192	1,207	533	407	29	589	2,234	8,145	48	918	428	1,207	1,454
Plums, prunes	5,600	2,240	861	285	69	582	2,800	3,270	567	329	717	986	1,047
Grapes, raisins	8,009	2,002	904	297	61	886	2,503	92	921	0	370	294	633
Nuts:													
Almonds	516	464	230	287	777	342	395	0	177	0	360	328	290
Pecans	128	102	60	32	235	22	49	.2	115	5	14	14	55
Walnuts	912	730	348	319	1,278	154	261	10	477	58	98	117	312

[1] Average yields per acre as reported by the United States Census for selected periods.
[2] Computed by dividing the nutrient content of the food at retail by daily allowances of food nutrients for a moderately active man, as recommended by the National Research Council.

TABLE 24.—*Average outputs of farm products, food at retail, and food nutrients per 1,000 units of feed used to produce specified livestock products* [1]

Farm product and food use	Farm products	Food at retail	Number of days a moderately active man can be supplied with a daily allowance of each of the food nutrients [2]										
			Food energy	Protein	Fat	Calcium	Iron	Vitamin A	Thiamine	Ascorbic acid	Riboflavin	Niacin	Average of 10 nutrients
	Pounds	*Pounds*	*Days*	*Days*	*Days*	*Days*	*Days*	*Days*	*Days*	*Days*	*Days*	*Days*	*Days*
Dairy products:													
Milk, whole	819	799	83	181	188	535	20	115	8	64	311	27	153
Evaporated milk	819	383	80	174	183	528	26	139	56	26	312	23	155
Butter	819	40	45	2	198	4	3	121	---	0	1	1	38
Cheese, American	819	81	48	126	158	402	18	129	11	0	93	5	99
All dairy products [3]	819	454	67	113	189	228	14	120	48	35	319	16	115
Dairy enterprise [4]	819	---	54	101	156	236	29	83	43	24	140	61	93
Poultry:													
Chicken enterprise [5]	179	---	33	125	94	34	125	103	45	8	80	68	72
Eggs	172	174	37	128	108	47	156	159	54	0	117	3	81
Chickens	172	151	27	121	70	8	66	0	26	23	10	187	54
Broilers	191	168	30	134	78	9	74	0	29	25	12	208	60
Turkeys	146	133	35	116	108	6	100	0	26	21	10	180	60
Hogs:													
Pork and lard	215	152	116	82	486	5	82	0	46	0	45	231	109
Pork	---	120	73	82	291	5	82	0	46	0	45	231	86
Lard	---	32	44	0	195	0	0	0	0	0	0	0	24

See footnotes at end of table.

TABLE 24.—*Average outputs of farm products, food at retail, and food nutrients per 1,000 units of feed used to produce specified livestock products* [1]—Continued

Farm product and food use	Farm products	Food at retail	Number of days a moderately active man can be supplied with a daily allowance of each of the food nutrients [2]										
			Food energy	Protein	Fat	Calcium	Iron	Vitamin A	Thiamine	Ascorbic acid	Riboflavin	Niacin	Average of 10 nutrients
	Pounds	*Pounds*	*Days*	*Days*	*Days*	*Days*	*Days*	*Days*	*Days*	*Days*	*Days*	*Days*	*Days*
Cattle:													
All beef cattle	130	63	21	60	69	3	53	0	25	0	26	134	39
Fattening cattle	103	50	17	48	55	2	42	0	20	0	21	107	31
Sheep:													
All sheep	50	24	9	19	32	1	21	0	28	0	14	29	15
Fattening lambs	104	51	17	48	55	2	42	0	20	0	21	108	31

[1] A unit of feed is defined as the quantity of feed equivalent to 1 pound of corn. The outputs shown do not include an allowance for byproducts such as skim milk, whey, and tankage which indirectly are sources of food or for nonfood byproducts such as wool and hides. The farm value of these byproducts expressed as percentages of the total farm value of all the products derived from the farm product in the 1943–45 period are as follows: milk for butter—10, milk for cheese—4, beef cattle—17, sheep—29, and hogs—1.

[2] Computed by dividing the nutrient content of the food at retail by daily allowances of food nutrients for a moderately active man, as recommended by the National Research Council.

[3] All milk used for dairy products as in the 1943–45 period.

[4] Includes cull cows, veal calves, and all milk used as in the 1943–45 period.

[5] Includes chickens and eggs in the combination they were produced in the 1943–45 period.

TABLE 25.—*Food produced from feed used to increase milk production per cow and to increase weights of hogs and beef cattle*

Increased feeding to increase production	Additional food output per 100 feed units		
	Edible products	Protein	Fat
MILK PRODUCTION PER COW [1]			
	Pounds	*Pounds*	*Pounds*
From 6,438 to 7,517 pounds	160	5. 6	6. 4
From 7,517 to 8,317 pounds	125	4. 4	5. 0
From 8,317 to 8,915 pounds	97	3. 4	3. 9
From 8,915 to 9,366 pounds	80	2. 8	3. 2
From 9,366 to 9,708 pounds	65	2. 3	2. 6
From 9,708 to 9,971 pounds	54	1. 9	2. 2
MARKET WEIGHT OF HOGS [2]			
From 150 to 175 pounds	15. 2	1. 2	9. 6
From 175 to 200 pounds	15. 4	1. 1	10. 7
From 200 to 225 pounds	15. 4	. 8	11. 6
From 225 to 250 pounds	15. 4	. 6	12. 6
From 250 to 275 pounds	15. 2	. 4	13. 3
From 275 to 300 pounds	14. 8	. 2	14. 0
YEARLING STEERS [3]			
From 640 to 740 pounds	10. 3	1. 1	4. 9
From 740 to 840 pounds	9. 9	1. 0	5. 2
From 840 to 940 pounds	9. 7	. 9	6. 2
From 940 to 1,040 pounds	9. 0	. 7	5. 7
From 1,040 to 1,140 pounds	7. 5	. 5	5. 3

[1] Computed from JENSEN (*12, p. 80*), milk-producing capacity of the cows reported upon in these experiments is much greater than the average for all cows in the United States, but response in milk production to heavier feeding probably is representative.   Data reporting feeding practices on Wisconsin farms show that the rate of concentrate feeding is not continued to the point where 1 pound of additional feed concentrates returns less than 1 pound of milk.   Over a period of 15 years an increase of 1 pound of concentrates was accompanied by an average increase of 1.17 pounds of milk.   See GILBERT (*9, pp. 19–27*).

[2] Computed from ATKINSON and KLEIN (*1, p. 19*).

[3] Computed from NELSON (*22, p. 31*).

TABLE 26.—Average outputs of farm products, food at retail, and food nutrients per 8-hour day of farm labor used to produce specified livestock products [1]

Farm product and food use	Farm products	Food at retail	Number of days a moderately active man can be supplied with a daily allowance of each of the food nutrients [2]										
			Food energy	Pro-tein	Fat	Cal-cium	Iron	Vita-min A	Thia-mine	Ascorbic acid	Ribo-flavin	Niacin	Average of 10 nutri-ents
	Pounds	Pounds	Days	Days	Days	Days	Days	Days	Days	Days	Days	Days	Days
Dairy products:													
Milk, whole	218	213	22	48	50	142	5	31	23	17	83	7	43
Evaporated milk	218	102	21	46	49	140	7	37	15	7	83	6	41
Butter	218	11	12	---	52	1	1	32	---	0	---	---	10
Cheese, American	218	22	13	34	42	107	5	34	3	0	25	1	26
All dairy products [3]	218	121	18	30	50	90	4	32	13	9	50	4	30
Dairy enterprise [4]	218	---	18	33	51	80	9	28	14	8	47	17	30
Poultry:													
Chicken enterprise [5]	46	---	9	36	26	9	34	27	12	3	21	22	20
Eggs	46	45	9	33	28	12	41	41	14	0	30	1	21
Chickens	58	51	9	41	24	3	22	0	9	8	4	63	18
Broilers	61	54	10	43	25	3	24	0	9	8	4	66	19
Turkeys	29	26	7	23	22	1	20	0	5	4	2	36	12
Hogs:													
Pork and lard	96	68	52	36	217	2	37	0	199	0	20	103	67
Pork	---	54	32	36	130	2	37	0	199	0	20	103	56
Lard	---	14	20	0	87	0	0	0	0	0	0	0	11

Cattle:													
All beef cattle	109	53	18	51	58	3	44	0	21	0	23	113	33
Fattening cattle	55	27	9	26	29	1	22	0	11	0	11	57	17
Sheep:													
All sheep	52	25	9	20	33	1	22	0	29	0	15	30	16
Fattening lambs	38	18	7	15	24	1	16	0	21	0	11	22	12

[1] The 8 hours of farm labor includes labor to produce crops fed to livestock as well as direct labor on livestock. Average yields for crops and labor requirements in the 1941–45 period were used. The outputs of food shown do not include an allowance for the byproducts of food such as skim milk, whey, and tankage which indirectly are a source of food or for the nonfood products such as wool and hides. The farm value of these byproducts expressed as percentages of the total farm value of all the products derived from the farm product are as follows: milk for butter—10, milk for cheese—4, beef cattle—17, lamb products—29, and hogs—1.

[2] Computed by dividing the nutrient content of the food at retail by daily allowances of food nutrients for a moderately active man, as recommended by the National Research Council.

[3] Milk used as in the 1943–45 period.

[4] Includes cull cows, veal calves, and milk used as in the 1943–45 period.

[5] Includes chickens and eggs in the combination produced in the 1943–45 period.

TABLE 27.—*Average outputs of farm products, food at retail, and food nutrients per 8-hour day of farm labor used to produce specified food crops* [1]

Farm product and food use	Farm products	Food at retail	Number of days a moderately active man can be supplied with a daily allowance of each of the food nutrients [2]										
			Food energy	Protein	Fat	Calcium	Iron	Vitamin A	Thiamine	Ascorbic acid	Riboflavin	Niacin	Average of 10 nutrients
	Pounds	*Pounds*	*Days*	*Days*	*Days*	*Days*	*Days*	*Days*	*Days*	*Days*	*Days*	*Days*	*Days*
Grain:													
Barley, pearl barley	1,073	590	319	314	36	54	447	0	216	0	109	554	205
Buckwheat, flour	364	204	110	83	14	13	76	0	192	0	37	130	66
Corn, yellow cornmeal	583	416	231	245	93	42	427	194	566	0	156	259	221
Corn, cornflakes	583	219	119	113	9	12	82	0	105	0	42	105	59
Oats, oatmeal	904	373	223	344	166	114	732	0	619	0	117	129	244
Rice, white	567	374	198	185	6	19	100	0	60	0	22	157	75
Rice, brown	567	448	242	218	46	99	210	0	398	0	50	618	188
Rye, light flour	588	448	243	258	24	45	153	0	203	0	69	122	112
Rye, whole flour	588	556	303	404	57	193	118	0	790	0	261	292	242
Wheat, white flour	1,231	874	470	613	47	94	383	0	174	0	66	204	205
Wheat, whole flour	1,231	1,207	656	1,016	146	262	1,439	0	2,035	0	338	2,035	793
Other staple food crops:													
Beans, dry edible	300	264	140	377	23	221	1,030	0	477	28	141	169	261
Peas, split peas	1,322	1,124	602	1,785	68	465	2,548	38	2,953	135	731	285	961
Potatoes, Irish	941	875	95	96	51	46	197	12	233	753	66	257	181
Sweetpotatoes	340	293	48	29	10	43	66	1,759	72	336	34	54	245
Peanuts, peanut butter	88	50	47	85	146	21	36	0	30	0	18	246	63
Soybeans, whole edible	747	672	356	1,521	737	773	2,033	66	2,321	0	471	423	870
Sugar beets, gran. sugar	2,334	343	208	0	0	0	14	0	0	0	0	0	22
Sugarcane, gran. sugar	1,943	147	87	0	0	0	6	0	0	0	0	0	9
Sugar beets, brn. sugar	2,334	366	212	0	0	158	360	0	0	0	0	0	73
Sugarcane, brn. sugar	1,943	158	90	0	0	68	154	0	0	0	0	0	31

Oil-bearing crops:												
Cottonseed	35	5	68	0	30	0	0	0	0	0	0	10
Peanuts	88	24	33	0	146	0	0	0	0	0	0	18
Soybeans	747	105	143	0	637	0	0	0	0	0	0	78

[1] 1941–45 average yields and labor requirements per acre were used. The outputs shown do not include an allowance for the value of byproducts or joint products such as feeds which indirectly are a source of food and for the nonfood products. The farm value of these byproducts expressed as percentages of the total farm value of all the products derived from the farm product in the 1943–45 period are as follows: corn for cornflakes—63, corn for corn meal—20, wheat for white flour—25, wheat for whole wheat flour—7, wheat for macaroni—60, rice—24, sugar beets for sugar—7, sugarcane for sugar—4, cotton for oil—88, peanuts for oil—31, and soybeans for oil—58.

[2] Computed by dividing the nutrient content of the food at retail by daily allowances of food nutrients for a moderately active man, as recommended by the National Research Council.

TABLE 28.—*Average outputs of farm products, food at retail, and food nutrients per 8-hour day of farm labor used to produce specified vegetables* [1]

Farm product and food use	Farm products	Food at retail	Number of days a moderately active man can be supplied with a daily allowance of each of the food nutrients [2]										
			Food energy	Protein	Fat	Calcium	Iron	Vitamin A	Thiamine	Ascorbic acid	Riboflavin	Niacin	Average of 10 nutrients
	Pounds	*Pounds*	*Days*	*Days*	*Days*	*Days*	*Days*	*Days*	*Days*	*Days*	*Days*	*Days*	*Days*
Fresh vegetables:													
Asparagus	126	115	4	12	1	11	30	78	42	173	33	30	41
Beans, lima	245	226	18	43	4	32	78	24	67	174	29	26	50
Beans, snap	232	206	12	29	2	69	77	106	43	218	42	35	63
Beets	613	552	28	43	2	63	157	9	41	251	47	52	69
Cabbage	2,214	1,882	59	123	17	358	267	102	289	4,341	198	112	587
Cantaloups	460	391	6	7	2	17	29	570	31	360	16	44	108
Carrots	550	494	29	34	8	97	132	4,747	89	158	64	66	542
Cauliflower	339	292	6	21	1	16	54	11	40	549	32	23	75
Celery	1,976	1,779	37	94	14	318	207	0	107	474	107	107	146
Cucumbers	685	588	9	19	2	23	49	0	48	212	83	20	46
Eggplant	949	826	30	51	9	61	110	17	148	209	91	176	90
Lettuce	1,586	1,285	24	70	10	111	171	439	171	411	135	43	158
Onions	992	853	59	73	10	146	149	36	86	433	42	34	107
Peas, green	224	212	15	42	2	12	69	59	103	154	40	60	56
Peppers, green	685	616	23	41	7	33	77	297	111	3,756	52	58	445
Spinach	430	348	10	43	5	131	325	2,440	102	1,017	156	61	429
Sweet corn	1,074	924	57	84	26	19	69	125	166	246	112	147	105
Tomatoes	464	348	11	20	5	19	69	304	55	431	28	59	100
Watermelons	945	822	18	12	4	16	28	204	55	142	45	22	55

Canned vegetables:													
Asparagus	252	172	6	18	3	20	65	94	33	153	33	42	47
Beans, green lima	255	364	39	90	7	56	234	43	38	175	40	54	78
Beans, snap	278	376	11	24	0	58	200	141	35	90	41	38	64
Beets	1,711	568	34	37	0	48	128	10	19	159	37	19	49
Cabbage for kraut	2,994	2,305	69	164	28	602	441	23	215	2,459	1,049	153	520
Peas, green	1,023	1,457	152	321	35	208	995	720	467	758	189	399	424
Spinach	991	1,070	40	159	26	547	651	6,596	64	941	203	100	933
Sweet corn	1,872	702	81	91	21	16	135	129	51	225	74	178	100
Tomatoes	1,341	586	19	38	7	37	133	560	90	588	44	125	164

[1] 1936–45 average yields and labor requirements were used.
[2] Computed by dividing the nutrient content of the food at retail by daily allowances of food nutrients for a moderately active man as recommended by the National Research Council.

TABLE 29.—*Average outputs of farm products, food at retail, and food nutrients per 8-hour day of farm labor used to produce specified fruits* [1]

Farm product and food use	Farm products	Food at retail	Number of days a moderately active man can be supplied with a daily allowance of each of the food nutrients [2]										
			Food energy	Protein	Fat	Calcium	Iron	Vitamin A	Thiamine	Ascorbic acid	Riboflavin	Niacin	Average of 10 nutrients
	Pounds	Pounds	Days	Days	Days	Days	Days	Days	Days	Days	Days	Days	Days
Fresh fruit:													
Apples	273	246	21	4	5	7	25	18	25	59	10	16	19
Apricots	200	182	15	11	1	15	32	434	16	36	16	39	62
Avocados	144	131	39	11	157	6	22	25	37	94	34	32	46
Grapefruit	896	851	38	18	7	54	64	12	63	1,373	26	34	169
Grapes	226	203	22	10	5	19	44	13	33	46	12	26	23
Lemons	417	396	16	14	9	19	10	0	34	671	2	11	79
Limes	135	128	8	5	1	8	3		14	161	2	4	21
Oranges	595	565	31	23	5	76	61	70	94	1,221	22	30	163
Peaches	303	270	18	8	1	11	54	190	15	112	26	65	50
Pears	357	321	28	12	6	20	29	6	17	69	26	11	22
Plums	302	269	22	12	3	25	49	81	113	72	18	43	44
Blueberries	58	57	6	2	2	5	17	15	5	56	8	5	12
Strawberries	37	33	2	2	1	5	10	2	3	115	5	3	15
Cranberries	67	64	6	5	3	13	22	19	5	91	10	6	18
Raspberries	35	31	3	2	2	6	11	9	3	44	4	3	9
Dried fruit:													
Apples, nuggets	273	27	16	2	2	4	42	0	5	18	5	4	10
Apricots	200	39	17	13	1	19	72	263	1	30	14	39	47
Plums, prunes	302	121	47	15	4	31	151	177	31	18	38	53	56
Grapes, raisins	226	56	25	8	2	25	70	3	26	0	10	8	18
Nuts:													
Almonds	31	28	14	17	47	21	24	0	11	0	22	20	18
Pecans	26	20	12	6	47	4	10	0	23	1	3	3	11
Walnuts	81	65	31	28	113	14	23	1	42	5	8	10	28

[1] National average labor requirements and average yields as reported by United States Census.
[2] Computed by dividing the nutrient content of the food at retail by daily allowances of food nutrients for a moderately active man, as recommended by the National Research Council.

TABLE 30.—*Average outputs of farm products, food at retail, and food nutrients per unit of all farm resources used to produce specified livestock products* [1]

Farm product and food use	Farm products	Food at retail	Number of days a moderately active man can be supplied with a daily allowance of each of the food nutrients [2]										
			Food energy	Protein	Fat	Calcium	Iron	Vitamin A	Thiamine	Ascorbic acid	Riboflavin	Niacin	Average of 10 nutrients
	Pounds	*Pounds*	*Days*	*Days*	*Days*	*Days*	*Days*	*Days*	*Days*	*Days*	*Days*	*Days*	*Days*
Dairy products:													
Milk, whole	221	215	22	49	51	144	5	31	23	17	84	7	43
Evaporated milk	316	147	31	67	71	203	10	54	22	10	120	9	60
Butter	446	22	24	1	108	2	2	66	0	0	1	1	20
Cheese, American	348	34	21	54	67	171	8	55	5	0	40	2	42
All dairy products [3]	288		23	39	67	115	5	42	16	12	63	5	39
Dairy enterprise [4]			23	44	60	74	11	32	19	12	64	21	36
Poultry:													
Chicken enterprise [5]			7	29	22	8	29	24	10	2	18	16	16
Eggs	40	39	8	29	24	11	35	36	12	0	26	1	18
Chickens	40	36	6	28	17	2	16	0	6	5	2	44	13
Broilers	35	31	4	24	14	2	13	0	5	5	2	38	11
Turkeys	30	27	7	24	22	1	21	0	5	4	2	37	12
Hogs:													
Pork and lard	74	53	40	28	168	2	28	0	154	0	16	80	52
Pork		42	15	28	101	2	28	0	154	0	16	80	43
Lard		11	25	0	67	0	0	0	0	0	0	0	9
Cattle:													
All beef cattle	82	40	14	38	43	2	33	0	16	0	17	84	25
Fattening cattle	58	28	10	27	31	1	24	0	11	0	12	60	18
Sheep: All lamb products	97	47	17	37	61	2	41	0	54	0	28	56	30

[1] A unit of all farm resources is defined as the quantity of resources required to produce $10 worth of the farm product in the 1943–45 period. The value of the farm product is the adjusted farm value obtained by deducting value of byproducts and adding Government payments to the gross farm value.
[2] Computed by dividing the nutrient content of the food at retail by daily allowances of food nutrients for a moderately active man, as recommended by the National Research Council.
[3] All milk used as in the 1943–45 period.
[4] Includes cull cows, veal calves, and milk used as in the 1943–45 period.
[5] Includes chickens and eggs in the combination produced in the 1943–45 period.

TABLE 31.—*Average outputs of farm products, food at retail, and food nutrients produced per unit of all farm resources used to produce specified food crops* [1]

| Farm product and food use | Farm products | Food at retail | Number of days a moderately active man can be supplied with a daily allowance of each of the food nutrients [2] | | | | | | | | | | |
			Food energy	Protein	Fat	Calcium	Iron	Vitamin A	Thiamine	Ascorbic acid	Riboflavin	Niacin	Average of 10 nutrients
	Pounds	*Pounds*	*Days*	*Days*	*Days*	*Days*	*Days*	*Days*	*Days*	*Days*	*Days*	*Days*	*Days*
Grain:													
Barley, pearl barley	578	318	172	169	19	29	241	0	117	0	59	299	110
Buckwheat, flour	526	295	158	120	20	18	111	0	277	0	53	187	94
Corn, yellow corn meal	629	449	248	265	101	46	460	209	611	0	168	278	239
Corn, cornflakes	735	276	150	141	12	16	103	0	132	0	54	83	74
Oats, oatmeal	578	238	143	219	107	73	468	0	395	0	75	82	156
Rice, white	296	195	104	96	4	10	52	0	31	0	12	82	39
Rice, brown	296	195	105	95	20	43	407	0	173	0	21	270	113
Rye, light flour	602	459	248	265	25	47	226	0	208	0	71	125	122
Rye, whole flour	602	570	311	414	59	197	1,035	0	809	0	268	300	339
Wheat, white flour	538	382	205	267	21	41	95	0	76	0	29	89	82
Wheat, whole flour	538	527	287	444	64	114	759	0	889	0	148	889	359
Other staple food crops:													
Beans, dry edible	172	152	80	217	14	128	593	0	275	16	81	97	150
Peas, split peas	213	181	97	287	11	75	410	61	475	22	118	166	172
Potatoes, Irish	402	374	40	41	2	20	84	5	100	319	28	110	75
Sweetpotatoes	264	227	37	23	8	33	51	1,363	56	260	26	42	190
Peanuts, peanut butter	122	70	65	118	201	29	50	0	41	0	25	341	87
Soybeans, whole edible	303	273	145	618	299	352	826	27	943	0	191	171	357
Sugar beets, gran. sugar	1,786	262	158	0	0	0	11	0	0	0	0	0	17
Sugarcane, gran. sugar	3,704	278	173	0	0	0	12	0	0	0	0	0	18
Sugar beets, brown sugar	1,786	280	162	0	0	121	276	0	0	0	0	0	56
Sugarcane, brown sugar	3,704	278	172	0	0	129	293	0	0	0	0	0	59

Vegetable fats:													
Margarine	120	120	133	5	56	1	9	217	0	0	0	0	42
Salad and cooking oil	116	116	157	0	700	0	0	0	0	0	0	0	86
Vegetable shortening	101	101	138	0	611	0	0	0	0	0	0	0	75

[1] A unit of all farm resources is defined as the quantity of resources required to produce $10 worth of the farm product in the 1943–45 period. The value of the farm product is the adjusted farm value obtained by deducting value of the byproducts and adding Government payments to farmers to the gross farm value.

[2] Computed by dividing the nutrient content of the food at retail by daily allowances of food nutrients for a moderately active man, as recommended by the National Research Council.

TABLE 32.—Average outputs of farm products, food at retail, and food nutrients per unit of all farm resources used to produce specified vegetables [1]

Farm product and food use	Farm products	Food at retail	Number of days a moderately active man can be supplied with a daily allowance of each of the food nutrients [2]										
			Food energy	Protein	Fat	Calcium	Iron	Vitamin A	Thiamine	Ascorbic acid	Riboflavin	Niacin	Average of 10 nutrients
	Pounds	Pounds	Days	Days	Days	Days	Days	Days	Days	Days	Days	Days	Days
Fresh vegetables:													
Asparagus	95	87	3	9	1	8	22	59	31	131	26	23	31
Beans, lima	103	94	8	18	2	14	33	10	29	73	12	11	21
Beans, snap	126	112	6	16	1	37	42	57	24	118	23	19	34
Beets	666	599	31	46	2	69	170	10	44	272	51	56	75
Cabbage	551	468	15	30	4	89	66	26	72	1,080	49	29	146
Cantaloups	203	172	3	13	1	8	13	251	14	159	7	20	48
Carrots	390	351	20	25	5	69	94	3,374	63	113	45	47	386
Cauliflower	223	192	4	13	1	11	35	8	27	360	21	15	50
Celery	214	192	4	10	2	34	22	0	11	51	12	12	16
Cucumbers	194	167	3	5	1	7	14	0	13	60	24	6	13
Eggplant	186	167	6	10	2	12	22	3	29	41	18	35	18
Kale	253	205	10	33	5	168	110	901	48	917	104	33	233
Lettuce	238	193	4	10	2	17	26	66	26	62	20	6	24
Onions	334	287	20	25	3	49	50	12	29	145	14	12	36
Peas, green	131	124	9	24	1	7	40	35	60	90	23	35	32
Peppers, green	124	108	4	7	1	6	14	52	19	656	9	10	78
Spinach	204	166	5	20	2	62	155	1,161	49	484	74	29	204
Sweet corn	262	225	14	20	6	4	17	30	40	60	26	36	25
Tomatoes	172	129	4	7	2	7	26	113	21	160	10	21	37
Watermelons	613	533	12	8	3	10	18	132	35	92	30	14	35

Canned vegetables:												
Asparagus	120	82	3	9	2	9	31	45	16	73	16	20	22
Beans, green lima	176	123	14	30	2	19	79	15	13	59	14	18	26
Beans, snap	199	269	8	17	0	42	143	101	25	65	30	27	46
Beets	980	325	19	21		28	73	5	11	91	21	11	28
Cabbage for kraut	1,196	1,554	47	111	18	406	298	15	145	1,658	707	103	351
Peas, green	240	342	36	75	8	49	234	169	109	178	44	93	100
Spinach	398	370	14	55	9	189	225	2,284	22	326	70	35	323
Sweet corn	1,060	398	46	52	12	9	76	73	29	127	42	101	57
Tomatoes	731	320	10	21	4	20	72	305	49	320	24	68	89

¹ A unit of all farm resources is defined as the quantity of resources required to produce $10 worth of farm products in the 1943–45 period.

² Computed by dividing the nutrient content of the food at retail by daily allowances of food nutrients for a moderately active man as recommended by the National Research Council.

TABLE 33.—*Average outputs of farm products, food at retail, and food nutrients per unit of all farm resources used to produce fruits* [1]

Farm product and food use	Farm products	Food at retail	Number of days a moderately active man can be supplied with a daily allowance of each of the food nutrients [2]										
			Food energy	Protein	Fat	Calcium	Iron	Vitamin A	Thiamine	Ascorbic acid	Riboflavin	Niacin	Average of 10 nutrients
	Pounds	*Pounds*	*Days*	*Days*	*Days*	*Days*	*Days*	*Days*	*Days*	*Days*	*Days*	*Days*	*Days*
Fresh fruit:													
Apples	189	170	15	3	4	5	17	12	17	41	7	11	13
Apricots	126	115	9	7	1	10	20	274	10	23	10	24	39
Avocados	69	63	19	5	75	3	10	12	17	45	16	15	22
Grapefruit	329	312	14	7	3	20	23	4	23	504	10	13	62
Grapes	209	188	20	9	5	18	41	12	30	43	12	24	21
Lemons	278	264	11	9	6	13	7	0	23	448	2	7	53
Limes	140	133	8	5	1	8	3	0	14	167	2	4	21
Oranges	323	307	17	13	3	41	33	38	51	663	12	16	89
Peaches	122	109	7	3	1	4	22	77	6	45	10	26	20
Pears	148	133	12	5	3	8	12	2	7	28	10	4	9
Plums	132	117	9	5	1	11	22	35	49	31	8	19	19
Strawberries	46	42	2	2	1	6	12	2	3	145	6	4	18
Dried fruit:													
Apples, nuggets	338	34	20	3	0	5	52	0	5	23	6	5	12
Apricots	31	6	3	2	0	3	11	41	0	5	2	6	7
Plums, prunes	98	39	15	5	1	10	49	57	10	6	12	17	18
Grapes, raisins	106	26	12	4	1	12	33	1	12	0	5	4	8
Nuts:													
Almonds	27	25	12	15	41	18	21	0	9	0	19	17	15
Pecans	35	28	16	9	64	6	13	1	31	1	4	4	15
Walnuts	42	34	16	15	59	7	12	0	22	3	4	5	14

[1] A unit of all farm resources is defined as the quantity of resources required to produce $10 worth of the farm product in the 1943–45 period.

[2] Computed by dividing the nutrient content of the food at retail by daily allowances of food nutrients for a moderately active man, as recommended by the National Research Council.

TABLE 3'.—Average outputs of farm products, food at retail, and food nutrients per unit of all farm and nonfarm resources used to produce specified livestock products [1]

Farm product and food use	Farm products	Food at retail	Number of days a moderately active man can be supplied with a daily allowance of each of the food nutrients [2]										
			Food energy	Protein	Fat	Calcium	Iron	Vitamin A	Thiamine	Ascorbic acid	Riboflavin	Niacin	Average of 10 nutrients
	Pounds	Pounds	Days	Days	Days	Days	Days	Days	Days	Days	Days	Days	Days
Dairy products:													
Milk, whole	140	137	14	31	32	92	3	20	15	11	53	5	28
Evaporated milk	174	81	17	37	39	112	5	30	12	5	66	5	33
Butter	339	17	19		82	2	1	50	0	0	0	1	16
Cheese, American	220	22	13	34	43	108	5	34	3	0	25	1	27
All dairy products [3]	182		15	24	42	73	3	27	10	7	40	3	24
Dairy enterprise [4]			14	28	38	45	7	2	12	7	41	13	21
Poultry:													
Chicken enterprise [5]			6	21	16	6	21	18	7	1	14	10	12
Eggs	31	30	6	22	18	8	27	27	9	0	20	1	14
Chickens	27	24	4	19	11	1	10	0	4	4	2	29	8
Broilers	23	20	4	16	9	1	9	0	4	3	1	25	7
Turkeys	19	17	5	15	14	1	13	0	3	3	1	24	8
Hogs:													
Pork and lard	51	36	27	19	115	1	19	0	105	0	11	55	35
Pork		28	17	19	69	1	19	0	105	0	11	55	29
Lard		8	10	0	46	0	0	0	0	0	0	0	6
Cattle:													
All beef cattle	56	28	9	26	30	1	23	0	4	0	12	58	16
Fattening cattle	40	20	7	19	22	1	17	0	8	0	8	42	12
Sheep: All lamb products	60	29	11	23	38	2	25	0	34	0	17	34	18

[1] A unit of all farm and nonfarm resources is defined as the quantity of all farm and nonfarm resources required to make available $10 worth of the food product at retail in the 1943–45 period. The value of the food product is the adjusted retail value obtained by adding Government payments to producers and processors and deducting processing taxes from retail value or price.

[2] Computed by dividing the nutrient content of the food at retail by daily allowances of food nutrients for a moderately active man, as recommended by the National Research Council.

[3] All milk used for dairy products as in the 1943–45 period.

[4] Includes cull cows, veal calves, and all milk used as in the 1943–45 period.

[5] Includes chickens and eggs in the combination they were produced in the 1943–45 period.

TABLE 35.—*Average outputs of farm products, food at retail, and food nutrients per unit of all farm and nonfarm resources used to produce specified food crops* [1]

Farm product and food use	Farm products	Food at retail	Number of days a moderately active man can be supplied with a daily allowance of each of the food nutrients [2]										Average of 10 nutrients
			Food energy	Protein	Fat	Calcium	Iron	Vitamin A	Thiamine	Ascorbic acid	Riboflavin	Niacin	
	Pounds	*Pounds*	*Days*	*Days*	*Days*	*Days*	*Days*	*Days*	*Days*	*Days*	*Days*	*Days*	*Days*
Grain:													
Barley, pearl barley	236	130	70	69	8	12	99	0	48	0	24	122	45
Buckwheat, flour	220	124	66	50	8	8	46	0	116	0	22	78	39
Corn, yellow corn meal	265	189	104	111	42	19	193	88	257	0	71	117	100
Corn, cornflakes	199	75	41	38	3	4	28	0	36	0	15	36	20
Oats, oatmeal	253	104	62	96	47	32	205	0	173	0	33	36	68
Rice, white	128	85	45	42	2	4	23	0	14	0	5	36	17
Rice, brown	107	85	46	41	9	19	176	0	75	0	9	117	49
Rye, light flour	226	172	93	99	9	18	85	0	78	0	27	47	46
Rye, whole flour	182	172	94	125	18	60	313	0	245	0	81	91	103
Wheat, white flour	243	172	93	121	9	19	43	0	34	0	13	40	37
Wheat, whole flour	176	172	94	145	21	37	249	0	291	0	48	291	118
Other staple food crops:													
Beans, dry edible	110	97	51	139	9	82	379	0	175	10	52	62	96
Peas, split peas	125	106	57	169	6	44	241	36	279	13	69	98	101
Potatoes, Irish	234	217	24	24	1	11	49	3	58	186	16	64	44
Sweetpotatoes	126	109	18	11	4	16	24	653	27	125	13	20	91
Peanuts, peanut butter	58	33	31	56	96	14	24	0	20	0	12	163	42
Soybeans, whole edible	93	83	44	188	91	107	252	8	288	0	58	52	109
Sugar beets, gran. sugar	861	127	74	0	0	0	5	0	0	0	0	0	8
Sugarcane, gran. sugar	1,773	133	80	0	0	0	6	0	0	0	0	0	9
Sugar beets, brown sugar	806	133	73	0	0	55	124	0	0	0	0	0	25
Sugarcane, brown sugar	1,656	133	77	0	0	72	131	0	0	0	0	0	28

Vegetable fats:											
Margarine	0	42	47	2	208	0	3	76	0	0	0	34
Salad and cooking oil	0	33	45	0	199	0	0	0	0	0	0	24
Vegetable shortening	0	42	57	0	255	0	0	0	0	0	0	31

[1] A unit of all farm and nonfarm resources is defined as the quantity of all farm and nonfarm resources required to make available $10 worth of the food product at retail in the 1943–45 period. The value of the food product is the adjusted retail value obtained by adding Government payments to producers and processors and deducting processing taxes from retail prices.

[2] Computed by dividing the nutrient content of the food at retail by daily allowances of food nutrients for a moderately active man, as recommended by the National Research Council.

TABLE 36.—*Average outputs of farm products, food at retail, and food nutrients per unit of all farm and nonfarm resources used to produce specified vegetables* [1]

Farm product and food use	Farm products	Food at retail	Number of days a moderately active man can be supplied with a daily allowance of each of the food nutrients [2]										
			Food energy	Protein	Fat	Calcium	Iron	Vitamin A	Thiamine	Ascorbic acid	Riboflavin	Niacin	Average of 10 nutrients
	Pounds	*Pounds*	*Days*	*Days*	*Days*	*Days*	*Days*	*Days*	*Days*	*Days*	*Days*	*Days*	*Days*
Fresh vegetables:													
Asparagus	48	44	1.5	4.5	0.5	4.0	11.0	29.5	15.5	65.5	13.0	11.5	15.6
Beans, lima	54	49	4.2	9.4	1.0	7.3	17.3	5.2	15.2	38.2	6.3	5.8	11.0
Beans, snap	66	59	3.1	8.4	.5	19.4	22.0	29.8	12.6	61.7	12.0	9.9	17.9
Beets	180	162	8.4	12.4	.5	18.6	45.9	2.7	11.9	73.4	13.8	15.1	20.3
Cabbage	211	180	5.7	11.7	1.5	33.9	25.3	9.8	27.5	413.9	18.8	10.9	55.9
Cantaloups	55	46	.8	.8	.3	2.2	3.5	67.8	3.8	42.9	1.9	5.4	12.9
Carrots	149	134	7.8	9.4	2.0	26.1	35.9	1,285.8	24.2	42.9	17.2	17.9	146.9
Cauliflower	60	52	1.1	3.5	.3	3.0	9.4	2.2	7.3	97.2	5.7	4.0	13.4
Celery	58	52	1.1	2.7	.5	9.2	5.9	2.2	3.0	13.8	3.2	3.2	4.3
Cucumbers	52	45	.8	1.4	.3	1.9	3.8	0	3.5	16.2	6.5	1.6	3.6
Eggplant	50	44	1.6	2.7	.5	3.2	5.9	.8	7.8	11.1	4.9	9.4	4.8
Kale	101	82	4.0	13.2	2.0	67.2	44.0	360.4	19.2	366.8	41.6	13.2	93.2
Lettuce	113	91	1.9	4.7	.9	8.0	12.3	31.2	12.3	29.3	9.5	2.8	11.3
Onions	151	130	8.9	11.2	1.3	22.4	22.8	5.4	13.0	65.7	6.3	5.4	16.2
Peas, green	52	50	3.6	9.6	.4	2.8	16.0	14.0	24.0	36.0	9.2	14.0	13.0
Peppers, green	50	43	1.6	2.8	.4	2.4	5.6	20.8	7.6	262.4	3.6	4.0	31.1
Spinach	108	88	2.6	10.5	1.1	32.7	81.7	611.8	25.8	255.1	39.0	15.3	107.6
Sweet corn	104	89	5.6	8.0	2.4	1.6	6.8	12.0	16.0	23.6	10.4	14.4	10.1
Tomatoes	68	51	1.6	2.8	.8	2.8	10.4	44.8	8.4	63.6	4.0	8.4	14.8
Watermelons	166	144	3.2	2.2	.8	2.7	4.9	35.6	9.4	24.8	8.1	3.8	9.6

Canned vegetables:												
Asparagus	36	25	.9	2.7	.6	2.7	9.3	13.5	4.8	21.9	4.8	6.0	6.7
Beans, green lima	54	38	4.2	9.3	.6	5.7	24.3	4.5	3.9	18.0	4.2	5.4	8.0
Beans, snap	59	80	2.4	5.0	0	12.5	42.8	30.3	7.4	19.3	8.9	8.0	13.7
Beets	196	65	3.8	4.2	0	5.6	14.6	1.0	2.2	18.2	4.2	2.2	5.6
Cabbage for kraut	295	384	11.5	27.5	4.5	100.2	73.5	3.8	35.8	409.0	174.5	25.5	86.6
Peas, green	61	86	9.1	19.0	2.0	12.4	59.2	42.8	27.6	45.0	11.1	23.5	25.2
Spinach	120	112	4.2	16.5	2.7	57.0	67.8	688.2	6.6	98.1	21.0	10.5	97.3
Sweet corn	191	72	8.3	9.4	2.2	1.6	13.7	13.1	5.2	22.9	7.6	18.2	10.2
Tomatoes	180	79	2.4	5.1	1.0	4.9	17.7	75.1	12.2	78.7	5.8	16.8	22.0

[1] A unit of all farm and nonfarm resources is defined as the quantity of resources required to produce $10 worth of the food product at retail in the 1943-45 period.

[2] Computed by dividing the nutrient content of the food at retail by daily allowances of food nutrients for a moderately active man, as recommended by the National Research Council.

TABLE 37.—*Average outputs of farm products, food at retail, and food nutrients per unit of all farm and nonfarm resources used to produce fruits* [1]

Farm product and food use	Farm products	Food at retail	Number of days a moderately active man can be supplied with a daily allowance of each of the food nutrients [2]										
			Food energy	Protein	Fat	Calcium	Iron	Vitamin A	Thiamine	Ascorbic acid	Riboflavin	Niacin	Average of 10 nutrients
	Pounds	Pounds	Days	Days	Days	Days	Days	Days	Days	Days	Days	Days	Days
Fresh fruit:													
Apples	100.2	90.1	8.0	1.6	2.1	2.6	9.0	6.4	9.0	21.7	3.7	5.8	7.0
Apricots	50.4	46.0	3.6	2.8	.4	4.0	8.0	109.6	4.0	9.2	4.0	9.6	15.5
Avocados	27.6	25.2	7.6	2.9	30.0	1.2	4.0	4.8	6.8	18.0	6.4	6.0	8.7
Grapefruit	134.9	127.9	5.7	2.9	1.2	8.2	9.4	1.6	9.4	206.6	4.1	5.3	25.4
Grapes	83.6	75.2	8.0	3.6	2.0	7.2	16.4	4.8	12.0	17.2	4.8	9.6	8.6
Lemons	114.0	108.2	4.5	3.7	2.5	5.3	2.9	0	9.4	183.7	.8	2.9	21.6
Limes	57.4	54.5	3.3	2.0	.4	3.3	1.2	0	5.7	68.5	.8	1.6	8.7
Oranges	146.3	139.1	7.7	5.9	1.4	18.6	14.9	17.2	23.1	300.3	5.4	7.2	40.2
Peaches	48.8	43.6	2.8	1.2	.4	1.6	8.8	30.8	2.4	18.0	4.0	10.4	8.0
Pears	59.2	53.2	4.8	2.0	1.2	3.2	4.8	.8	2.8	11.2	4.0	1.6	3.6
Plums	52.8	46.8	3.6	2.0	.4	4.4	8.8	14.0	19.6	12.4	3.2	7.6	7.6
Strawberries	18.4	16.8	.8	.8	.4	2.4	4.8	.8	1.2	58.0	2.4	1.6	7.3
Dried fruit:													
Apples, nuggets	173.4	17.4	10.3	1.5	1.0	2.6	26.7	0	2.6	11.8	3.1	2.6	6.2
Apricots	15.9	3.1	1.5	1.0	0	1.6	5.6	21.0	0	2.6	1.0	3.1	3.7
Plums, prunes	50.3	20.0	7.7	2.6	.5	1.5	25.1	29.2	5.1	3.1	6.2	8.7	9.3
Grapes, raisins	54.4	13.3	6.2	2.1	.5	6.2	16.9	.5	6.2	0	2.6	2.1	4.3

[1] A unit of all farm and nonfarm resources is defined as the quantity of resources required to produce $10 worth of the food product at retail in the 1943–45 period.

[2] Computed by dividing the nutrient content of the food at retail by daily allowances of food nutrients for a moderately active man, as recommended by the National Research Council.

World Food Supply

An Arno Press Collection

Agricultural Production Team. **Report on India's Food Crisis & Steps to Meet It.** 1959

Agricultural Tribunal of Investigation. **Final Report.** Presented to Parliament by Command of His Majesty. 1924

Bennett, M. K. **The World's Food:** A Study of the Interrelations of World Populations, National Diets and Food Potentials. 1954

Bhattacharjee, J. P., editor. **Studies in Indian Agricultural Economics.** 1958

Brown, Lester R. **Increasing World Food Output:** Problems and Prospects. 1965

Brown, Lester R. **Man, Land & Food:** Looking Ahead at World Food Needs. 1963

Christensen, Raymond P. **Efficient Use of Food Resources in the United States.** Revised Edition. 1948

Crookes, William. **The Wheat Problem.** Revised Edition. 1900

Developments in American Farming. 1976

Dodd, George. **The Food of London.** 1856

Economics and Sociology Department, Iowa State College. **Wartime Farm and Food Policy,** Pamphlets 1-11. 1943/44/45

Edwards, Everett E., compiler and editor. **Jefferson and Agriculture:** A Sourcebook. 1943

Famine in India. 1976

Gray, L. C., et al. **Farm Ownership and Tenancy.** 1924

Hardin, Charles M. **Freedom in Agricultural Education.** 1955

High-Yielding Varieties of Grain. 1976

[India] Famine Inquiry Commission. **Report on Bengal.** 1945

Johnson, D. Gale. **Forward Prices for Agriculture.** With a New Introduction. 1947

King, Clyde L., editor. **The World's Food.** 1917

Marston, R[obert] B[right]. **War, Famine and our Food Supply.** 1897

Mosher, Arthur T. **Technical Co-operation in Latin-American Agriculture.** 1957

The Organization of Trade in Food Products: Three Early Food and Agriculture Organization Proposals. 1976

Projections of United States Agricultural Production and Demand. 1976

Rastyannikov, V. G. **Food For Developing Countries in Asia and North Africa:** A Socio-Economic Approach. Translated by George S. Watts. 1969

Reid, Margaret G. **Food For People.** 1943

Schultz, Theodore W., editor. **Food For the World.** 1945

Schultz, Theodore W. **Transforming Traditional Agriculture.** 1964

Three World Surveys by the Food and Agriculture Organization of the United Nations. 1976

U. S. Department of Agriculture, Agricultural Adjustment Administration. **Agricultural Adjustment:** A Report of Administration of the Agricultural Adjustment Act, May 1933 To February 1934. 1934

U. S. Department of Agriculture. **Yearbook of Agriculture, 1939:** Food and Life; Part 1: Human Nutrition. 1939

U. S. Department of Agriculture. **Yearbook of Agriculture, 1940:** Farmers in A Changing World. 1940

[U. S.] House of Representatives, Committee on Agriculture. **Oleomargarine.** 1949

[U. S.] National Resources Board. **Report of the Land Planning Committee. Part II.** 1934